Sex, Drugs and Walking Sticks

MIRROR BOOKS

Copyright © Dr Miriam Stoppard

The right of Dr Miriam Stoppard to be identified as the owner of this work has been asserted in accordance with the Copyright, Designs and Patents Act, 1988. All Rights Reserved.

No part of this publication may be reproduced, stored in a retrieval system, or transmitted in any form, or by any means, electronic, mechanical, photocopying, recording or otherwise without the prior permission in writing of the copyright holders, nor be otherwise circulated in any form of binding or cover other than in which it is published and without a similar condition being imposed on the subsequent publisher.

1

Written with Alison Phillips

First published in hardback in Great Britain and Ireland in 2026 by Mirror Books, a Reach PLC business.

www.mirrorbooks.co.uk
@TheMirrorBooks

ISBN: 9781917439596
eBook ISBN: 9781917439602

Every effort has been made to trace copyright.
Any oversights will be rectified in future editions.

Editing and Production: Christine Costello, Roy Gilfoyle
Cover Design: Chris Collins, Julia Mans

Printed and bound by CPI Group (UK) Ltd,
Croydon, CR0 4YY.

Sex, Drugs and Walking Sticks

A GUIDE TO LIVING YOUR BEST LIFE
IN YOUR 60s, 70s, 80s AND BEYOND

Dr Miriam Stoppard

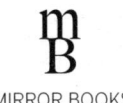

MIRROR BOOKS

This book is designed to be a guide to many aspects of later life and potential health issues but if you are concerned about a medical condition or symptoms please always discuss these with your doctor

For my wonderful WhatsApp group of Witches and Bitches: Joan, Ilana, Nicole, Barbara, Judy, Marion, Sandi and Caroline

Contents

Author's Note 11

A

Alcohol 14
Anaemia 17
Appetite 20
Armd (Age-Related Macular Degeneration) 22
Arthritis 24

B

Back – Taking Care Of 29
Balance & Unsteadiness 30
Bereavement 34
Blood Pressure (BP) 37

C

Cancer 42
Cannabis (Medical) 45
Caring For A Loved One 47
Cataracts 49
Concentration 50
Cosmetic Surgery 52
Covid Boosters 55

D

Dating (Online) 57
Dementia/Alzheimer's 60
Depression 66
Divorce 74
Driving 78
Drugs/Medications 79
Dry Eyes, Dry Mouth 85

E

Eating 88
Exercise Is Everything 92

F

Falls 97
Family 100
Fitness – How Fit Are You? 103
Fractures 106
Future Fears 107

G

Gardening 111
Giddiness 112
Girlfriends – I Don't Know What I'd Do Without Them 113
Glaucoma 118
Gout 119
GPs 121
Grandparenting 124

H

Hair	131
Health Checks – Essential	136
Heartburn	137
High Heels	139
Hormones	141
Hypothermia	146

I

IBS	148
Incontinence	149
Inheritance	151

J

Joy	153

K

K – Potassium	156

L

Living Will	158
Loneliness	160

M

Make-Up	166
Masturbation, Vibrators & Orgasms	171
Microbiome	174
Mindfulness	177
Money Worries	179

N

Norovirus	183

O

Optimism	186
Osteoporosis	190

P

Pain & Pain Management	195
Parkinson's Disease	197
Pedicures	198
Pets	200
Posture	202
Prostate Gland	205
Protein	207
Pulse	210

Q

Quads	213

R

Reading	215
Remarriage & New Partnerships	217
Resting	219
Retirement	220

S

Sex… It Never Stops	224
Shere Hite	239
Shingles	241

Single Again, Why Would I Not Want To Be?	242	**W**	
Sleep	244	Walk…	287
Smoking	248	Walking Sticks	288
Snoring/Sleep Apnoea	251	Warning Signs You Must Never Ignore	290
Social Media	253	Weight	291
Strength	254	Weight Loss Drugs	295
Stress	255	Work	295
Stretching	259	Wrinkles	297
Sugar – Beware!	262	**X**	
Superagers	264		
Supplements	265	Xerostomia, Dry Mouth	299
Swimming	269	Xerophthalmia, Dry Eyes	299
T		**Y**	
Thirst	271		
Tiredness	273	Yoga	300
Travel	275	**Z**	
U			
UV Skin Protection	278	Zenith	302
V		Acknowledgements	304
Vaccination	281		
Viagra	282		
Vitamins	284		

Author's Note

HONESTLY, I DIDN'T FEEL LIKE I had another book in me. All through my life I've written about what was happening to my body in order to give women insight into what was happening to theirs. So, when I was having children, and given that all the baby books at that time were written by men, whereas I'd pushed out a couple, I felt I could write with some authority.

There followed half a dozen books on baby and childcare, also on child development. But what about before? So, Conception, Pregnancy and Birth. And what about dads? So, a book for dads followed. And then I got menopausal, so a book on menopause. I got a lump in my breast so a book on breast cancer. Then I was in my 50s so a health guide for people of my age. My publisher wanted a sex book and unable to resist an offer of work, a sex book appeared. I wrote books on all the TV series I made. Then, as I entered my 60s, grandchildren came along so I wrote a couple of books on becoming a grandparent. On and on…

So why *Sex, Drugs and Walking Sticks?* Well, from my long perspective of 88 years I've learned a lot about good health, the transition into getting older, keeping fit, looking after mental wellness, having grandchildren, and becoming widowed. The SEX in the title is to do with what I view as a lifetime of loving. Just because an erection isn't perfect and a vagina gets dry aren't reasons to forgo sex, albeit a different kind from younger times.

The DRUGS is in the title because as we get older and comorbidities arrive there are life-saving medicines we have to take daily to remain active and healthy. And the WALKING STICKS is there because I believe with the help of a walking stick one can, literally, still be active to the end of one's life. Metaphorically though, there's information throughout my book you can "lean on" and see it as a supportive walking stick for life in general.

It's been a fervent wish that my books, written mainly for women, will strengthen and fortify them to be active participants in decisions that affect their health. To give women the confidence to speak out for their medical rights and not to be put off by what can often feel like intimidating doctors and medical staff. So I see my books as giving women backbone, bottle.

The same goes for this one. As we get older, frailer, and less confident, ageing can become a series of setbacks to overcome. Well, my book is designed to give you an idea as to what lies ahead with advice on how to prepare, prevent or soften the impact of getting on.

One of the things I've learned is not to be taken for granted, to fight my corner – with a friend for moral support if necessary, to draw on our years of wisdom, to adjust to the fact that our bodies get older and weaker. If you're looking for bottle – confidence – this book can supply it. If you'd like some insight on what can work for you, I recount what, over the years, has worked for me.

What's the background to walking sticks? Well, as we get older and stiffer and weaker a walking stick can be a life-saver. My favourite walking stick (a foldable one that can go in my handbag) has saved me from many a tumble. And despite hearing older people commonly see a stick as an admission of approaching decrepitude, I see it as a tool that keeps me going.

In fact my walking stick is key to my life and my determination to be an active participant in life, rather than an observer as I get older. Fortunately, as my fitness has improved I find I resort to my walking stick less often than I used to, in fact not at all for the last year.

Sex, Drugs & Walking Sticks

The truth is, my walking stick gives me bottle, the bottle to go outdoors, ever more important as we get older and our confidence ebbs. It makes me feel confident enough to stride out and walk till I'm tired. I live in Central London but luckily within half a mile of a huge park. My favourite walk is to follow paths that crisscross the park, stopping to admire the amazing trees. I feel uplifted for the whole walk.

But that's not the full story on walking sticks. Honestly, this book is full of walking sticks, metaphorically speaking. The way I see it is you can use the information I give you as a means of supporting your life in your golden years, encouraging you to be the best you can be. In other words acting like a "walking stick". You'll find them scattered through my book, often in the form of hints and tips.

Just a note of explanation, for ease of reference, I'm going to take you through the things that can affect your later life alphabetically, so we start with A and Alcohol.

A

Alcohol

AS YOUR LIVER AGES, YOUR heart ages and your brain ages too, so drinking alcohol will have a greater and greater effect on your body. It can't be metabolised as quickly as when you were younger so your hangover will be worse.

You may find that your doctor says a couple of glasses of red wine now and then is good for you because it makes you feel relaxed and that's helpful to your heart. Next time you are visiting your doctor be sure to ask what they think is a suitable level for any conditions you may have. Most people won't say no to a glass of champagne on a special occasion but if you're like me and find that alcohol starts to disagree with you as you've become older, I think that's the signal to stop.

When I was pregnant with my first child in the early 1970s we didn't know how alcohol affected a pregnant woman's body, that came quite a bit later. I was sitting with some friends in a restaurant and I had a glass of wine. Suddenly I found myself unable to sit up and I slipped from my chair onto the floor. I was drunk on one glass of wine because the pregnancy hormones disabled my liver and my blood alcohol levels soared. Pregnant women can't metabolise alcohol efficiently so levels rise quickly and dangerously. Now I recommend that alcohol is an absolute no-no during pregnancy. Always remember alcohol is a poison and it really taxes the ageing liver to get rid of it. While your blood levels are high every organ in your body is affected by it and if those organs aren't 100% they'll be functioning well below par.

Here are my top tips to safe drinking in older age:

- As you get older it's important to try to keep to NHS recommended limits which say men and women shouldn't drink more than 14 units a week on a regular basis. A small (125ml) glass of wine is 1.5 units. A pint of higher strength (5.2%) lager, beer or cider is 3 units.
- Eating something before you drink, even a biscuit, can help ameliorate a hangover, which is just as well as hangovers get worse as we get older.
- Do drink twice as much water as alcohol, and a big glass of water before bed to avoid dehydration which can be a particular problem in older age as we drink less water.
- Do eat food as you drink to soak up the alcohol.
- Always sip alcohol rather than gulp it.
- Don't mix drink and sex – you're more careless and could catch an STD which is on the rise in the 60+ age group.
- Don't binge and drink a week's allowance in a short time; it's bad for your liver.
- Don't mix drink and drugs, you won't be able to handle an emergency.
- Stay off alcohol for a few days after a party to let your liver recover.
- Do a drink-free weekend once a month.
- Don't drink and drive and never ride in a car driven by someone who's been drinking.

The real problem comes if you are frequently drinking too much. Alcohol is almost as bad for you as smoking. It can greatly harm your body and several major organs like the heart, the liver and the kidneys if you overindulge.

In England in 2022, the number of units consumed by all people over 16 years of age in an average week was 13.3[1], in Scotland it was 12.6 units on average[2], and in Wales about 9.74 units per week[3].

Across the United Kingdom, a significant number of adults regularly drink over the Chief Medical Officers' low-risk guidelines: e.g. in England 32% of men and 15% of women, in Northern Ireland 25% of men and 9% of women[4], in Scotland 31% of men and 15% of women and in Wales 25% of men and 10% of women.

So at what point should you be worried that your drinking has reached a problem stage?

You need answer yes only to one of these questions to mean alcohol is affecting your life and you should be thinking of seeking help from your doctor or Alcoholics Anonymous.

- Has a friend or family member close to you said they're worried about your drinking?
- When faced with a problem, do you turn to alcohol as a crutch?
- Does your drinking affect work or your relationships?
- Have you ever promised to stop drinking and failed?
- Have you ever tried to stop drinking and had distressing physical or psychological symptoms?

---

1   https://digital.nhs.uk/data-and-information/publications/statistical/health-survey-for-england/2022-part-1/health-survey-for-england-2022-part-1-data-tables
2   https://www.gov.scot/publications/scottish-health-survey-2022-volume-1-main-report/pages/10/
3   https://www.gov.wales/national-survey-wales-headline-results-april-2022-march-2023-html#126278
4   https://www.health-ni.gov.uk/publications/health-survey-northern-ireland-first-results-202324

- Have you ever had a blackout or total loss of memory while drinking?
- Have you ever needed to see a doctor because of drinking?

Alcoholism can lead to severe debilitating disease especially when the liver develops cirrhosis and chronic inflammation, brought about by alcohol, a poison. Unless drinking stops, cirrhosis is fatal.

If you want to control your drinking there are various successful approaches. But have you checked out Alcoholics Anonymous? I'm convinced its 12 step programme and lifelong adherence is one of the best options.

Anaemia

ANY FORM OF ANAEMIA MEANS the oxygen-carrying power of the blood is lowered so all the tissues may go short of nourishment. It's always serious and particularly so in older people who may have comorbidities like heart disease and high blood pressure, because anaemia may make the two conditions worse.

There are two main kinds of anaemia that affect us as we get older. The first, and by far the most common, is iron-deficiency anaemia where the body, and primarily the red blood cells, are low on iron. This usually means that iron is being lost from the body almost always in a form we can't see like bleeding from the gut. It may occur as part of malabsorption syndrome where iron isn't being properly absorbed from food. In iron-deficiency anaemia, the iron in red blood cells is diminished and they can't therefore carry oxygen efficiently around the body to where it's needed. This shortage of iron in red blood cells shows as shortness of breath, even when not exercising, palpitations, dizziness, paleness of the skin, and sometimes chest pain. A tell-tale sign of iron deficiency anaemia is spoon-shaped fingernails so they're concave instead of convex.

Before iron-deficiency anaemia can be treated the cause has to be found. It may be due to bleeding from the gastrointestinal tract (GIT) because of hiatus hernia, peptic ulceration, diverticulosis and occasionally haemorrhoids. Bleeding can occur from the stomach caused by the action of certain drugs, particularly aspirin and other NSAIDs (non-steroidal anti-inflammatory drugs) used for the treatment of conditions such as arthritis. This loss of blood from the GIT is in tiny quantities and only when it's cumulative does anaemia develop. Any cancer of the GIT may also lead to anaemia due to loss of blood.

If you're thought to have iron-deficiency anaemia, the first test is to look for hidden blood in your stool, "occult blood". Your GP can arrange for this and if it reveals a condition that needs treatment it will be arranged. Iron-deficiency anaemia responds dramatically to iron supplements, in the first instance, taken as tablets. A course of iron tablets taken for three to four months usually clears up any kind of iron-deficiency anaemia. Your doctor will probably want to keep an eye on you in case it should recur and you need further investigation and treatment.

The second type of anaemia seen in old age is called pernicious anaemia and it's due to a failure to absorb vitamin B12 from your food by the small intestine. About one in 10 patients who go to see their GP because of anaemia, have pernicious anaemia. This is quite different from iron-deficiency anaemia and affects the production of red blood cells in the bone marrow which slows down without vitamin B12. The result is there are too few red blood cells available to keep the body ticking over. Characteristically in pernicious anaemia there are immature red cells circulating in the blood and these can be spotted by examining a blood sample under a microscope, confirming the diagnosis of pernicious anaemia. There are some telltale signs of pernicious anaemia such as sores at the corners of the mouth and a smooth tongue.

Patients sometimes complain that iron tablets upset them with nausea and indigestion, sometimes constipation and sometimes slight diarrhoea. You can lessen side effects by always making sure you take iron tablets after food. If you inform your doctor about these side effects, it's possible to change to an iron tablet that has fewer of these side effects. You can also get iron by injection, given into a muscle. If your iron-deficiency is extremely severe, you might be taken into hospital to have a blood transfusion to bump up your red blood cells. With pernicious anaemia you'll need to have injections of vitamin B12 periodically throughout your life, starting with quite a heavy loading dose of several injections in a month and then going on to a regime where you may only need an injection every two months. Your progress will be monitored through blood counts and your doctor will decide how often you need the B12 injections.

Besides affecting the blood, shortage of B12 also causes damage to the nervous system. A condition called peripheral neuropathy may occur with numbness and tingling in the fingertips and the toes. Besides the injections, it would be a good idea to eat food which is rich in vitamin B12 and these would be all animal products including eggs, dairy, meat, fish and shellfish. Vegetables themselves don't contain vitamin B12 though you may be able to obtain vegetable products that are enriched with it.

If you have any symptoms of anaemia please don't resort to self-treatment with iron tablets you may get from the pharmacy because it may not be iron that you need. You must see your doctor for a blood test which examines all the different elements in your blood that may contribute to anaemia.

Dr Miriam Stoppard

Appetite

OUR APPETITE TENDS TO DECREASE as we get older, our stomach capacity is less so we feel fuller sooner. And it can seem a great effort to prepare food if we're feeling tired. As we age, our metabolic rate slows down and so we require fewer calories. Also if we're less active our appetite is less because calories aren't being burned as they once were. With age, taste and smell can be blunted, making food less appetising. Swallowing may become uncomfortable too or even painful with certain foods.

Surprisingly, being underweight is more of a problem than being overweight in older people. A lot of medical conditions causing weight loss and problems like iron and vitamin deficiency are more common in the elderly. Medications can also sometimes lead to weight loss.

It is, however, essential to keep eating a balanced diet to maintain energy. As a woman you can aim for 1,500 calories a day and as a man 2,000 on average.

If you're feeling your appetite needs a bit of gingering up there are ways to increase your eating and enjoyment of food. For starters, you can create a step by step routine by choosing, preparing and cooking food yourself. Of course, this all begins with shopping. Perhaps you can make this more interesting by planning in advance what you would like to eat and looking out for some new ingredients.

Your interest in food may also be affected from having a dry mouth, something which is more and more common as we age. But don't accept it.

I have a dry mouth too and I prevent it by chewing gum. Before you eat, make sure your mouth is well-lubricated by sipping some water.

And if you really don't feel like cooking a meal, try finger foods such as crackers and cheese, pita bread and hummus, pâté and toast and eat all the healthy snacks you like. Don't miss an opportunity to eat if you feel like eating something. There are also all the drinkable meals such as soups, porridge and fruits, meal shakes or smoothies with fruits, vegetables and protein powder (which you can buy from pharmacies). If you find it hard to be enthusiastic about cooking a full meal, why not cook a family-sized meal then freeze what you don't eat for the following week?

The appetite can be blunted by constipation and nausea so if these are an issue you may need a doctor's help to treat both of them.

In general, concentrate on nutrient-dense, high-calorie foods. This is the one time that you can indulge yourself. Ice cream is good, so is chocolate, particularly dark chocolate. Peanut butter on toast is delicious, as is avocado with smoked salmon and any other fatty fish which you like.

It's not easy to make someone without an appetite eat but you can be supportive without being pushy. Smaller, more frequent meals often help. And it would be wise to avoid foods that have strong smells.

Here are my top tips for keeping your weight steady:

- Try to eat something at each meal. This doesn't mean you have to force yourself to finish or to overeat but try not to skip meals. Eat smaller portions more often if that feels better than one large meal.
- Try to set up a routine and eat meals at the same time every day. By having a routine you're less likely to forget to eat. It might help to put reminders on post-it notes in the kitchen.
- Eat wholegrains and lots of fruit and vegetables. Have a fruit bowl in the kitchen as a constant reminder.

- Eat healthy fats like olive oil, avocados, salmon and walnuts.
- And make sure you drink plenty of liquids during the day, say, 8-10 cupfuls.

ARMD (Age-Related Macular Degeneration)

LIKE THE REST OF THE body, our eyes age, and one of the most common conditions of late age is ARMD or, to give it its full name, age-related macular degeneration. The macula is the centre of the retina at the back of the eye where our vision is most vivid and detailed. ARMD usually affects people over 50 but can happen earlier. Macular disease is the primary cause of sight loss in the UK, with ARMD affecting around 700,000 people. The older we are, the greater our risk of developing the condition. Around one in every 200 people has ARMD at 60. However, by the age of 90 it affects one person in five[5].

It's rare for ARMD to cause total blindness, as it usually affects the central part of your vision. Nonetheless, reading and recognising faces may get more difficult. Our national treasure, the actor, Dame Judi Dench suffers from ARMD but it hasn't deterred her from working. At 90 years old her indomitable spirit prevails. I attended an event where we could watch her being sculpted and she admitted she might not be able to see the finished sculpture. Sad. Without treatment of ARMD your vision gets progressively worse, sometimes slowly over several years or more quickly, in a few weeks and months. We still don't know the cause, though many factors have been suggested, such

---

5   https://www.macularsociety.org/

as smoking, being overweight, high blood pressure and having a family history of ARMD.

ARMD causes inflammation in the macula where images of what we see pass through the optic nerves to the brain. Because of macular inflammation, the first symptom is often blurred or distorted vision in or near the centre of your vision and makes things like driving, watching TV, reading and recognising faces difficult. Your eyes may be sensitive to bright light and when you directly look at lights they may flicker and flash. Lines may look wavy or crooked and occasionally you may see things that aren't there.

So what should you look out for? Well, your eye may become red and painful and you have what's described as a dark curtain moving across your field of vision. Your vision may suddenly get worse and if any of these things happen, you should head to A&E immediately. Even better, go to the nearest eye hospital in your locality.

ARMD can be wet or dry, wet being the more serious of the two as it can worsen quickly, sometimes in days or weeks.

Dry ARMD usually progresses more slowly over several years. Another difference between the two is that treatment may be unnecessary for dry ARMD unless it develops into the wet form. With the wet form treatment is aimed at stopping vision getting worse and there are two main approaches to treatment. The first is an injection of medication directly into the eye and the second is light treatment aimed at destroying the bundles of blood vessels that cause wet ARMD. Do visit the Macular Society website https://www.macularsociety.org/ which has more information about all forms of ARMD and their treatments which are improving all the time.

If you have low vision there are things you can do to help yourself, such as using a magnifying glass to enlarge print. Make your lights brighter at home and there are software and mobile apps that can make your phone easier to use as well as your computer.

Dr Miriam Stoppard

Arthritis

I KNOW HOW LUCKY I AM not to suffer from arthritis and the pain it causes. Having painful joints can restrict all aspects of your life and having to cope with the chronic pain on a daily basis is exhausting. Living with any chronic disease, arthritis included, requires fortitude and a positive attitude to life. We know optimism helps. Someone who's optimistic can still take life at a tilt whereas a pessimist is disabled by their arthritis. Some people with chronic arthritis keep mobile and active. They do their own housework, ride bicycles and do the weekly shop.

There are two main types of arthritis, the first, *osteoarthritis* (OA) has been described as the natural ageing of joints through daily wear and tear. In the main it affects joints which are weight-bearing, so the hips and the knees are commonly affected. Over time the smooth cartilage that lines the joints becomes rough and uneven so the joint no longer works without friction. With age, these roughened surfaces not only make movement difficult, but cause great pain. OA is common, as shown by these stats from a 2023 NICE (National Institute for Health and Care Excellence) report[6].

- Approximately 10 million people (six million women, four million men) in the UK have OA, with an estimated 5.4 million people affected by knee OA and 3.2 million by hip OA.
- Approaching 350,000 people are diagnosed with OA each year.
- Symptoms start around 55 years.

---

6   https://cks.nice.org.uk/topics/osteoarthritis/background-information/prevalence/

- The frequency of OA cases rises sharply between 45–64 years of age, peaking at 75–84 years of age.

The second kind of arthritis, *rheumatoid arthritis* (RA), is an autoimmune condition where the body attacks the lining of the joints. In RA, however, it's not just the joints that are affected. Practically every organ in the body is affected in some way as the result of inflammation in collagen, the universal tissue that forms the scaffolding of most organs.

Living with rheumatoid arthritis is tough. But here is some advice which I hope proves helpful.

- Rest whenever you can because RA tires you out. Conserve your energy.
- Pay attention to your suppleness so after a bath or shower is a good time to do some mobility exercises such as step backwards and forwards with raised arms, rotate your body while you step backwards and forwards, arm circling, bridge against a wall, sideways tilting from the waist while standing. Don't do too much or your joints will ache, nor too little or your joints will stiffen.
- If your joints are sore the day after exercise you're doing too much. But move around normally as much as you can.
- Wearing hand splints at night is excellent for keeping your wrists and fingers aligned.
- Always take the drugs your doctor prescribes. Inform your doctor of any side effects. Drugs used for RA like DMD (disease modifying drugs) are powerful so talk to your doctor about them.
- Treatment for RA is long-term and necessary, improvement is slow.
- No need to cut out alcohol but drink in moderation.

Gout is a third kind of arthritis, which usually occurs in men and we think of it as being the result of high living – too much rich food and fine wine. It isn't always. It is caused by abnormal metabolism of protein which leads to the accumulation of uric acid in the blood. Needle-like crystals of uric acid are deposited in the joints, often in the big toe. It becomes extremely red, swollen and excruciatingly painful. During an attack some people find they can't even tolerate the weight of a sheet on the swollen joint.

It really is beneficial if you take care of your joints to keep them healthy, mobile and free of pain. You can destress your joints by not getting overweight and being conscious that all your weight eventually is borne by your knees and ankles. If you possibly can, put your joints through their full range of movements by keeping active. Anyone who walks every day, does their own household chores, and gardens a bit is already doing that.

It's also worth trying to protect your spine by paying attention to your posture. Protect your back when lifting something heavy by bending your knees and taking the pressure on your thighs rather than bending over and leveraging the comparatively weaker muscles of your back. Remember, fit, strong muscles protect your joints and strong abdominal muscles in your core act as a supportive splint for your spine, so make time to exercise your core and keep it strong.

Joint Replacements

Treating arthritis of the hip and knee with joint replacement is quite common nowadays. It didn't used to be. If you need one, a hip replacement will bring untold relief. Most are very successful and can give you a new lease of life. Soon you'll be astonished how active you can be again!

The operation replaces both the pelvic socket and the head of the thigh bone (femur) that fits into it. You'll probably need a general anaesthetic and after the op all that's necessary is a short stay in hospital and then you'll be able to go home.

Move slowly and carefully during the first two weeks post-op as the joint is unstable.

Over 100,000 hip replacements are being done in the UK each year most often for older people, whose joints may be arthritic, stiff and painful as the result of osteoarthritis. You might think about losing a bit of weight as preparation for your hip operation. Every kilo you lose is critical because when you walk your hip joint copes with stress equivalent to three to five times your body weight, rising to as much as 12 times your body weight during strenuous activity.

Immediately after surgery you lie on your back with your legs separated by a wedge-shaped cushion and after a few days you'll be able to walk using a Zimmer frame or crutches. Activity gradually returns and most people are able to drive after about eight weeks. A hip replacement operation can change your life and there's a 95% chance you'll have total freedom from pain and, in time, regain 75% of your normal range of movement.

Treating arthritis of the knee with joint replacement is also quite common now. It's done for osteoarthritis of the knees causing extreme pain and mobility problems.

The average age of knee replacement is 70 and it's done under general anaesthetic. After 2-3 weeks you'll be able to put some weight on the leg. Research says pain peaks at nine days post-op but the first week after the op is very painful. You should draw up an action plan with your doctor including pain management, regular physiotherapy, gentle increase in activity and lots of rest. The knee joint may seem stiff for a few months and high impact sports like jogging or skiing should be avoided. Stairs are difficult so avoid them. Cover the joint before showering to avoid infection.

Protecting your Knees

One way or another your knees take the brunt of bearing your weight, particularly if you gain weight. Add to that they can become affected by osteoarthritis due to normal wear and tear. The heavier you are the more severe the arthritis of your knees will be so it's worth looking after them all your life.

Exercises to Protect Your Knees

If you want to avoid knee replacement for your arthritic knee, strengthening your quads - they're the muscles at the front of your thighs - is essential. It could make you less likely to need replacement surgery. Each year in the UK, 100,000 people have to have a knee replaced because of arthritis but people who have strong quads are less likely to need a new knee. Strong quads reduce stress on the knee joint and improve the stability of the joint. How would you strengthen them? Walking each day helps, as does doing squats and lunges. But only attempt those if your balance is good and even then hang on to something.

Arthritis and Sex

It's possible for arthritis to affect your sex life because of stiffness and pain. For instance, the missionary position may be a no-no. Don't despair. Try a new position, such as the woman on the top which can be more comfortable. To ease pain, taking painkillers a couple of hours before sex is a good idea. Don't let problems with penetration put you off. There are many other options to choose from if you and your partner want to explore them. We all need physical closeness through touching and caresses. They bring comfort and reassurance. The "spoons" position is worth trying where one partner lies behind the other.

B

Back – Taking Care Of

BY THE TIME YOU REACH your 60s, your back has been subject to decades of wear and tear as the spine is one of the most overworked parts of the body.

Every day for 24 hours, including when you're asleep, your back is constantly stressed and strained. Having grandchildren can worsen any back problem because you'll want to lift them and hold them and your spine has to support you and them. But you can look after your back to minimise future wear and tear on your spine. Here's how:

- Don't bend down when you're doing something at floor level, such as weeding or playing with your grandchild. Kneel instead, it's easier on your back.
- Stooping and bending over puts a lot of strain on your joints and muscles, so just sit down.
- Remember to bend down from your knees not from your waist when lifting something heavy such as a child or a pushchair.
- Never carry anything at a distance from your body. Make sure you hold it close and bend from your knees when you put anything heavy down again.
- If you have to move something, don't face it and push with

your hands and shoulders, turn around and push with your back and bottom.
- Your core muscles, mainly your abdominal muscles which sit between your ribcage and pelvis, act as a splint for your spine and hold it steady, so keep them in good nick by pulling them in whenever you remember and count to five before letting them go.

Balance & Unsteadiness

MY BALANCE HAS NEVER BEEN that good, especially since my 50s. But even in my 40s it was dodgy. I remember I was doing a TV show with Terry Wogan called *The Health Show* and I was trying to demo balancing on one leg. I kept falling over so he had to catch me, to the merriment of the crew. My balance was just good enough up to my mid-70s (I skied until I was 73) but then I became steadily unsteady.

Trouble is, many parts of the body are involved in keeping us balanced and they act in unison. Their harmony is unconscious until something goes wrong when one part fails to function properly. Our balancing organ is in the inner ear and its job is to coordinate the constant stream of rapid fire messages that bombard it from the eyes, the muscles, the joints, and the feet. If your brain can't make sense of this disparate info, the balancing organ can't keep you balanced. This sophisticated, complicated system can go wrong, nearly always making you very dizzy. I've had two attacks of vertigo, both of which got better on their own but were deeply unpleasant. Even with my eyes closed the room wouldn't stop spinning and I couldn't stop being sick.

An ear doctor diagnosed the first one as *paroxysmal benign labyrinthitis* where parts of my actual balancing organ, the vestibular system, failed to function, something probably caused by a viral infection. The second, much more serious attack, overtook me in security at Toulouse Airport when I was travelling alone. From one second to the next I couldn't move, started to vomit and the room was spinning. Paramedics took me to A&E in France and from there I was admitted to hospital as an emergency. After days of exhaustive tests I was diagnosed as having *vestibular nerve inflammation* secondary to a virus (any virus) infection.

I was well enough to go home in a wheelchair five days later. My son, Ed, came to look after me and I have him to thank for my rapid recovery. He forced me to open my eyes till the vomiting stopped and he got me out of bed to walk the hospital corridors while I clung on to him. Both of my first and second attacks of vertigo can happen to anyone and if this happens to you I advise telling your doctor ASAP. When you've recovered enough to stand I'd recommend you see a *vestibular physiotherapist* who can diagnose exactly what's wrong with your balancing organ in your inner ear. In some cases they'll treat you with a head manoeuvre (Epley) and give you exercises to improve your balance.

But much of balance is down to ensuring strong legs and core muscles. So it's worthwhile encouraging core strength. A gentle local yoga or pilates class would help introduce you to planks and abbreviated push ups if you haven't done them before. Talk to your doctor first about what might help you. You might also want to attempt standing on one leg a couple of times each day – but only in a space where you can hang on to something to keep you steady and that's softly carpeted in case you fall. By far the best way to improve your leg strength and balance is to walk every day, with a stick if you need it and "spot" on an object in front of you.

And if you are concerned about your balance, always wear flat shoes and do a thorough sweep of your home each day to remove any potential trip-ups.

Improving your Balance

- As we get older good balance becomes more and more of a challenge as it can lead to falls and bone fractures. Start gently with 5-10 seconds of standing on one leg then switching to the other. In your 80s you only need to raise one foot a few inches off the ground. Once you've got the hang of it, increase the time you stand on one leg. A few seconds is better than nothing. Always make sure you have something to hang on to and carpet underfoot.
- Squats, not quite sitting down on a chair, are hard work but worth it because they're excellent for keeping your thighs (quads) and buttocks (glutes) strong. Holding your arms out in front of you, try sitting down till your bottom just touches the seat then stand up. Five reps are plenty to start with, then increase them.
- I find bird dog quite taxing. I have to think hard to alternate arms and legs but it's a superb balancing exercise. Once you're on all fours, stretch out your left arm and right leg at the same time while keeping your core muscles tight, then switch to the other arm and leg.

Small exercises to do all day long aid fitness, suppleness, mobility and strength

I have good days and bad days when my steadiness is good and not so good. I just see that as the normal rhythm of life.

We all want to remain strong, flexible and mobile as we get older but you don't need to take out a gym membership to achieve that. All you need to do are simple "corrections" throughout the day as and when you remember. Here is one of my favourites, especially on bad days when I feel a bit unsteady (when I feel like this I always take a walking stick when I go out). Indoors I use "spotting". This is what ballet dancers do so that they don't fall over when they stop spinning. You spot (fix your eyes) on something, anything – a picture, a door knob, a clock and you keep your eyes fixed on it as you walk.

Your brain loves this because it gives your balancing organ in your inner ear something steady to focus on and it keeps your eyes steady so that they send calm, visual messages about mobility to your brain. Then as I start to walk I go through a little ritual to help my body. I lower my shoulders, I draw my chin down and back and I engage my core muscles (my tummy in, back raised up). All this jogs your muscle memory and tones your muscles, your stability and your coordination.

Doing a gentle plank (on your knees and elbows) is really good for your core and upper body but I don't necessarily get down on the floor. In the bathroom I do leaning press ups on the basin (just four or five) and the same in the kitchen leaning on a surface. If I'm feeling really good I'll do a couple of yoga sun salutations.

Whenever I sit in an armchair I do ankle circling and I remind myself to get out of the chair without using my arms – essential to maintain your quads, your main walking muscles. I keep some weights (1kg) handy (a tin of beans is a good substitute) and I do forearm and upper arm raises (maybe ten) and just walk about my flat gently doing them.

One of the reasons we get unsteady as we get older is that we forget our feet. We forget how crucial they are for balance, particularly your big toe. Every time you walk remember your feet and give your balancing organ a treat. Feel your feet pressing into the ground first through your heel, then through the sole of your foot and then a big push through your big toe which is a powerful balancing organ.

The twisting movements of our hand and fingers get weaker as we age, as does grip strength. In fact you can tell a person's age by measuring their grip strength, which is largely down to the small muscles of your hands. As we age they shrink and weaken. A trick I've learned to keep them strong is to loosen a tight lid by holding the lid and pressing down, then unscrew. Most lids become free with this treatment and you keep your hand muscles strong.

Save your back by using your thighs. Every time you need to bend down for something, bend your knees to lower your upper body, keeping your back straight. So squat down, don't bend down. At first it may be a struggle to get back up from a squat but persist and help yourself with your arms. As your leg muscles strengthen you won't need to hang on to something to help yourself up.

I have a simple routine to stretch my neck muscles which I do in bed. Lying on a neck pillow I shuffle my hands and arms down the bed, keeping my head still and hold it maybe for 2-3 minutes. I concentrate on my breathing at the same time and slow it down. I'm usually ready for sleep when I release my arms.

Bereavement

MY HUSBAND DIED SUDDENLY, SO there was no time for preparation, foreseeing his loss, his absence, bolstering myself for the emotional turmoil, and putting in place some kind of support. For anyone in these circumstances the emotional turmoil is made worse by the immediate need to handle all the admin, and there's a surprising amount of that.

To those who are faced with bereavement, it becomes a phase of life that has to be endured just as we have to get through serious illness, our children leaving home or divorce. Grief accompanies most bereavements, but may be delayed by having to handle the immediate aftermath of a partner dying. Then it comes hammering in after a few weeks. Grief takes many forms and the classical stages of anticipation, sense of loss, numbness, anger, searching, denial, acceptance, letting go and regrowth but not always in these stages, and not always in this order. Grief is chaotic.

In terms of our life span, bereavement and the grief that comes with it, may be the hardest time we will ever live through.

Grieving is an individual matter. There's no right or wrong way to grieve, it's different for everyone, and different in many cultures for that matter. It's important to realise that grieving has to be got through somehow and it doesn't really matter how you manage to get it done. You should grieve exactly as you want to. For me it was opting out of life, staying on my own and I was overcome by apathy with no interest in anything that was going on around me.

Medically speaking grief has a different effect on women and men. During the first six weeks of bereavement, it's not uncommon for widowers to complain of heart trouble, which may go on to death from a "broken heart". Don't dismiss it, it's real. It's even written up in medical text books. Widows, on the other hand, tend to consult their doctors with gastric upsets and rheumatic conditions. Grief, with great sadness and sense of loss is often confused with depression. Food literally loses its taste and appetite goes. Sleep can be fitful, if at all. Guilt may creep in with personal recrimination for not having looked after your partner well enough. Asking yourself questions is inevitable. "How could I have prevented their death? Should I have taken better care of them, spent more time with them, talked to them more?" If you feel like crying, cry for days on end if you want to, if only because you're tending to your emotional needs. It's best not to make a concerted effort to forget, trying to forget means it will be all the more difficult to accept your partner has gone.

There are practicalities to be dealt with, such as telling your family doctor about the death which they can certify and issue a death certificate. The next stage is to *register* the death by taking the death certificate to the Registrar's office. You can, if you really want to, do all these things yourself, but I would strongly advise that you enlist the help of your family, in particular your children, to see to the statutory responsibilities of your partner's death, including funeral arrangements. Don't hesitate to ask your family doctor for their help and they'll always be sympathetic. I feel it's advisable to seek the help of your family if there's a *will* to be read and financial arrangements to be made. It's very tough doing this on your own and you shouldn't have to face it alone. No doubt relatives will try to persuade you to get in touch with friends. You should please yourself, but remember, one good friend may be enough to help you emerge from your despondency and take up the reins of life again. If you feel the need for the company of others and their comforting words, you might try drawing up a list of visits, short trips, holidays, stays with friends which might fill up the next few months. You could find looking forward to this re-entry into the outside world helps to soothe your grieving and gradually brings you back into the world.

Some thoughts to help you cope with bereavement:

- Give yourself enough space to grieve. Take no notice of people who are encouraging you to get back to normal. Once you feel like moving on, it's important for you to regain your identity or even possibly find a new one. Rather than continuing your past way of life, start doing some new things that really interest you.
- Defer big decisions. Don't make any until your grieving is over and you feel ready to get back to normal. Don't doubt yourself.

- Seek out an understanding person to whom you can talk about your feelings and bring a sense of perspective if you're overreacting or in a trough of self pity. When you can't see yourself pulling out of the depths of despair an objective point of view can really help.
- Your feelings and emotions during bereavement and grieving are legitimate and normal.
- Don't stay chained to the house, make sure you keep mobile by going out for walks and doing some shopping. If you have a car and feel like driving, get your friend to go with you once or twice a week to begin with to reacquaint yourself with driving and road conditions.
- Pay attention to your finances, keep them under control so that you don't suddenly find yourself in debt. Even if you've never done it before, it's a good idea to start budgeting your finances. If it's an unknown area, get a friend to show you how and start keeping a record of all your income and expenses. Try to balance the books at the end of each month.
- Eventually, you'll find that life goes on, and as a free agent, you're in the perfect position to take the holiday you always dreamed of. Make sure you look after yourself, give yourself the occasional treat and reward yourself with the trip of a lifetime.

Blood Pressure (BP)

YOUR BLOOD PRESSURE SHOULD BE normal to ensure good health. About 1 in 3 adults in the UK have high BP (hypertension), but many don't realise it. It's often called the "silent killer" because it has no symptoms but damages blood vessels and organs like the brain and kidneys nonetheless. A rise in blood pressure usually comes on in the older age groups caused by heart disease, furring up of the arteries with fat, weight gain and type 2 diabetes.

A high blood pressure can overwork your heart till it eventually loses strength. Over time a high BP can harm your heart, kidneys, brain, and eyes. Despite having no warning signs, it can lead to a heart attack and stroke. Excess weight or having a family history of high BP raises your risk for hypertension.

Because it usually has no symptoms, the only way to know for sure you have hypertension is to have your BP checked regularly by your doctor, especially if you have any of the above risk factors.

The good news is that high BP can be treated and often prevented.

It's normal for your BP to go up and down throughout each day because it's affected by the time of day, exercise, the food you eat, stress, and other factors. Problems can arise, though, if your BP stays too high for too long.

How to take your blood pressure

Taking your own blood pressure is reassuring. And, as it happens, when measured at home it's sometimes lower than when measured in a doctor's surgery where you may be anxious, suffering from what is often called "white coat syndrome" when there are too many medics around! Another advantage of taking your BP at home is that you can measure it three times then take an average. This has been shown to be the most reliable measurement of BP.

There are many cheap BP monitors you can buy on the internet or local pharmacy. Choose the simplest you can find that's reasonably priced. Make sure you get one with an explanatory leaflet on how to use it.

What's the normal range for your blood pressure?

Blood pressure is given as two numbers. The first number represents the pressure in your arteries as the heart pumps (systolic pressure). The second is the pressure as your heart relaxes and fills with blood (diastolic pressure). 120/80 is normal and as you get older it may rise to 140/90 which is considered acceptable. If you ever measure your blood pressure at home and you're higher than 140/90 make an appointment to see your doctor.

If you're diagnosed with high BP you and your doctor will agree a treatment plan. You'll likely be advised to move to a healthier lifestyle and to lose a bit of weight. You may also need to take medications, the dose being adjusted till your BP comes down to a normal level. Many people are on medication for high blood pressure but there are ways to help reduce it without the need for drugs.

Lowering your blood pressure without medication

Quit smoking

Now's the time to stop smoking because every cigarette you smoke increases your BP. Quitting smoking helps your BP return to normal.

Watch your waistline and lose weight

A high BP could drop somewhat with weight loss. The more weight you lose the greater the drop in BP. Just losing 10 pounds (4.5 kilograms) can help lower your BP.

Reduce salt (sodium) in your diet

Even a small reduction in salt can lower BP so choose low-sodium alternatives.

Lower your stress levels

Chronic stress contributes to high BP. Think about what causes you to feel stressed then consider how you can control or reduce stress.

Exercise regularly

It isn't a big ask. Just 30 minutes most days of the week can lower your BP but consistency is key, because if you stop, your BP may rise again.

Eat a healthy diet

By now you know what this is – a diet that is rich in wholegrains, fruits, vegetables and low-fat dairy products can help lower your BP. This eating plan is known as the Dietary Approaches to Stop Hypertension (DASH) diet[7].

Treatments for high blood pressure

There are different treatments and approaches to lowering high BP. Some of them, as I've said, don't use drugs at all but simply change lifestyle. Most doctors would like to start off treatment of high BP with some of these self-help measures if the BP isn't too high. They would start with changes to your diet as discussed above. For more information you can research the DASH approach which emphasises fruit, vegetables, low dairy, wholegrains and reduced saturated and total fat. It also encompasses a low salt intake so lowering your intake of sodium, and increasing your intake of calcium, magnesium and potassium. DASH stipulates increasing your physical activity and reducing your alcohol intake help to normalise your BP, as will stress management.

Minerals such as magnesium and potassium also help to normalise BP. Some products like dark cocoa (chocolate) and garlic boost nitric oxide and also causes blood vessels to relax and helps bring down your BP.

A good night's sleep would be a useful addition to this plan, as would tracking your BP at home so you can keep an eye on it. It's been shown that people who measure their BP every day have better control of it and adhere better to the non-drug approach

---

7   https://www.nhlbi.nih.gov/education/dash-eating-plan

to controlling high BP. As a precaution, refrain from eating too much of that delicious soft, black liquorice (yes, I mean it) as it is known to deplete your body of potassium, thereby raising your blood pressure. I fell foul of this and my blood pressure soared.

In terms of medicines used to treat BP, the first step would be taking water pills (diuretics). These drugs help remove sodium and water from the body, giving the heart less work to do.

Then there are two groups of drugs which are commonly used. The first is called ACE (Angiotensin-Converting Enzyme) inhibitors such as Ramipril and the second group ARBs (Angiotensin Receptor Blockers) such as Cozaar. ACE inhibitors act by relaxing blood vessels, and this relaxation causes the BP to drop. They do so by blocking hormones that constrict blood vessels.

And then there are calcium channel blockers such Amlodipine. It's used alone or together with other medicines. In addition, Amlodipine relieves angina (heart pain). As a calcium channel blocker it works by relaxing the blood vessels and lowering BP. This boosts the supply of blood and oxygen to the heart while reducing its workload. Pretty impressive, I'm sure you agree.

A new procedure for treating some kinds of high BP is the Simplicity Blood Pressure Procedure and involves threading a thin catheter through a blood vessel to reach the arteries near the kidneys. There, the nerve signals contributing to elevated blood pressure are interrupted. The catheter is then removed and no implant is left in the body.

C

Cancer

NO TWO CANCERS ARE THE same. In fact, there are as many cancers as there are people, even cancers within the same organ can be different, for example, there are different types of prostate cancer just as there are different types of breast cancer. This is because cancer is caused by gene mutations and there are literally millions of those. Cancer has always had bad press. "So and so died of cancer" was all that we heard within families and in the media. It was rare to hear, "So and so's treatment was successful and they're cured of cancer". At the present time, however, the progress in cancer research is so astounding there's good reason for optimism about the future. I certainly am optimistic.

Nonetheless, cancer accounts for about 1 in 6 deaths as we grow older and cases of many cancers, such as those of the lungs, the bowel and the skin, plus certain types of leukaemia and the prostate gland, rise with age.

Cancers can run in families and are inherited. The most well-known gene mutations which run in families and lead to cancer of the breast, ovary and colon cancer are called BRCA 1 and 2. Such gene mutations can be passed from generation to generation. Even though the BRCA genes cause two cancers in women they can also be carried by the men in her family and passed on to future generations of women and men. This kind of genetic inheritance can be tracked through a family tree and each individual member tested for it. As a result, cancer is no longer seen as a bogeyman. This improved awareness means that people will look out for early signs of cancer and consider changing their lifestyle in order to avoid it. And there's no doubt that changing your lifestyle will greatly help you to avoid getting cancer, including lowering the risk of cancers down to inherited mutations.

Most of these changes to lifestyle boil down to what you eat and how active you are. You can choose to eat a typically western diet which is high in UPFs (ultra processed foods), animal fat, sugar, salt and is loaded with calories. Or you can choose to eat what I would call a cancer-protective diet which would be rich in fibre and unprocessed carbohydrates such as in fruit and vegetables and wholegrains, plenty of low-fat dairy and short on red meat, avoiding as many processed foods as you can.

Having said that, I'm in favour of the 80/20 rule which I learned when I was in Stanford University, California, examining their heart health programme. The professor in charge of the programme said to me, "All you have to do is eat the right stuff 80% of the time and it hardly matters what you eat the other 20%". Ever since hearing that I've adhered to it. We also know that limiting your calorie intake will have a positive effect on protecting you from cancer, whereas the opposite applies to a calorie-heavy diet that results in being overweight. Obesity can participate in cancer formation and we have plenty of research on that[8].

The second way in which you can amend your lifestyle is to be more active. I feel I say this so often that I have actually started to bore myself. But it's true. Being active – and it doesn't have to be very active – will protect you against heart disease, stroke, high

---

8 https://www.cancer.gov/about-cancer/causes-prevention/risk/obesity/obesity-fact-sheet#:~:text=A%20study%20that%20used%20nationally,women%20(47%2C%2048)

blood pressure, obesity and cancers. There's no doubt about this. Again, there's lots of research to prove it[9]. If you're overweight/fat/obese, you not only have high levels of insulin you also have high levels of a cancer-causing hormone, insulin-like growth factor. You can really help yourself by having every cancer screening test that's offered to you and repeat them regularly. If you do that, the chances are that your cancer will be discovered early, when treatment has the best chance of a complete cure. An example of this is a girlfriend of mine, who had breast cancer some years ago when it was discovered to be small and treatment cured her. However, recently, a new cancer has formed which was discovered when it was less than the size of a pea because she has regular check-ups. This means her current treatment gives her a greater chance of a cure because the cancer was found so early.

Some cancers are more common as we get older, and this is simply because we live long enough for that cancer to develop. The good news is, as we're older, most of them are slow-growing and amenable to treatment. An example of this is chronic lymphatic leukaemia (CLL). It's a form of leukaemia that's most common in the elderly but if you had to have any leukaemia, CLL would be the one. It's what I would call a "gentle" cancer and can be treated with chemotherapy and immunotherapy. Nearly all cases go into remission and if they recur, another course of treatment will arrest the leukaemia. If you have CLL you're more likely to die with it rather than from it.

One of the reasons for optimism about cancer is that treatments are now very sophisticated. Our advanced technology treatments are often tailor-made or bespoke for individual cancers. By individual cancers I don't mean cancers of the prostate or cancers of the bowel. I mean each and every cancer of the prostate and each

---

9   https://evidence.nihr.ac.uk/alert/small-amounts-of-exercise-protect-against-early-death-heart-disease-and-cancer/

and every cancer of the bowel. This specific treatment stops one particular cancer in its tracks.

Latest treatments are fiendishly clever and have a high success rate. One of my favourites is immunotherapy where a person's immune system is alerted to the precise cancer they're suffering from. Furthermore, the immune system seeks out the particular DNA mutations which are causing the cancer and responds with specific antibodies that will attack those particular cancer cells. This to me is mind-boggling when you think of what we did in the past. Older treatments were like taking a hammer to crush a pea and made little distinction between the characteristics of individual cancers. Immunotherapy can be accompanied by chemotherapy if necessary. This two-pronged approach to treating cancer has revolutionised the way we tackle it and in some cases immunotherapy may be given as maintenance treatment after the cancer has been cured in order to prevent it from coming back.

Doctors do all they can to ameliorate cancer treatments but that doesn't mean that some of them aren't difficult to take. And some cancer patients are amazingly stoical. I've known many patients who suffer with each dose of chemotherapy but nonetheless are prepared to face the next one.

Cannabis (Medical)

IN THE UK CANNABIS IS now legal under certain circumstances. We can use medical cannabis for some forms of severe epilepsy, for the nausea and vomiting that occurs with some chemotherapy and for muscle stiffness and spasms in multiple sclerosis (MS). I remember way back in my television days, one of my researchers being diagnosed with MS. How she came to take her first dose of cannabis I don't know, but she found it very powerful in relieving painful muscle spasms. In those days cannabis was available only through an illegal route, from a drug dealer. She or her husband would go onto the street and find her cannabis illicitly. I was incensed by the unfairness of this and felt she ought to be able to have medical cannabis without the humiliation of seeking a drug dealer. She lobbied her local MP to have cannabis legalised for medical purposes and I supported her in her efforts but nothing came of it other than a few articles in newspapers.

Thank heavens the situation has changed now, at least somewhat. Medical cannabis which contains THC (psychoactive) and CBD (anti-inflammatory) can be used to relieve pain and chronic pain, though there's the danger of addiction if it's used in the long-term. Cannabis works by interacting with the ECS (endocannabinoid system) which plays a part in pain control, sleep and mood. Different forms of cannabis have different actions on the ECS. I must make it clear that cannabis containing THC is a controlled drug and possession is illegal except for personal and medical use. Medical cannabis is available on the NHS for the above conditions with a prescription from a specialist doctor. GPs can't prescribe medical cannabis. Cannabis in the form of cannabidiol (CBD) is legal and can be absorbed from under the tongue where it quickly passes into the bloodstream. CBD may stimulate serotonin receptors in the brain and so helps regulate your mood and may lower your anxiety and improve depression. Boots, Superdrug and some supermarkets sell CBD oil drops. The dose usually starts at 20 to 50 milligrams once a day.

I thought I should set out for you what you'd need to do to get a prescription for medical cannabis, bearing in mind that cannabis-based medicine can only be prescribed on the NHS by a specialist hospital doctor, or under a specialist's supervision, for a small number of patients, and these conditions might be considered.

- For epilepsy – if you (or your child) have one of the rare forms of epilepsy that might be helped by medical cannabis.
- For MS (multiple sclerosis) – if you have spasticity from MS and other treatments for this are not helping.
- For chemotherapy – if you are vomiting or feeling sick from chemotherapy and other anti-sickness treatments are not helping.

Before considering a cannabis-based product the specialist will discuss with you all the other treatment options first.

A prescription for medical cannabis would only be given when other treatments had failed or were not suitable, and if it was believed to be in your best interests.

Caring For A Loved One

IF YOU FIND YOURSELF IN the position of having to care for your partner or a family member you are joining a great band of people in the UK with a similar purpose. In fact, there are 5.7 million people providing unpaid care in the UK. Looking after a partner can be a full-time job, 24/7 with little respite, unless you ask other family members to give you a break. Some of us have had the role of full-time carer thrust upon us, for example, when a partner becomes seriously ill with a long-term condition such as motor neurone disease or if they start to develop dementia. Most of us, finding ourselves in this situation, would do whatever was necessary to keep life ticking over. Occasionally, with dementia which gradually gets worse, you'll be called upon to see to personal care such as bathing and dressing, making sure your partner can move around the house or flat safely, keeping appointments which may involve your driving, making travel arrangements, doing errands, grocery shopping, and the preparation of food. You may also have to carefully manage medication schedules and if medical needs become complicated to seek help from your GP.

There are many positive aspects of caring for a loved one. For instance, it means you may spend more time with your partner than you've done in the past, and that makes for a closer bond. Your partner may feel more comfortable with you than with a stranger and so is happier as a result. You may feel emotional satisfaction from being the helper which is good for your morale. And one of the most important aspects is, with you as the carer, the necessity to go into a care home may be avoided. In addition, a home carer is more cost-effective than a care home and you have control over any decisions which are made.

Then again, there are some downsides. Having experienced being a carer myself when my husband developed dementia, I know about the emotional strain it can bring in addition to the physical strain. You get very tired if you don't look after your personal needs, there's the possibility of burnout. You might regret the lack of free time and time for yourself. As your partner gets more sick and disabled you may have to give up an interesting job or work fewer hours. It's easy to feel isolated in this situation and resentment may creep in because you can't plan ahead. Get help from Home Care Services from your local council, or if the family will help you to pay, a private agency who will create a bespoke package for you.

Your partner's needs and preferences must be taken into consideration about you or anyone else being their carer. They may fear losing their independence, losing their dignity, and may go into denial about getting older and needing more care. They may also interpret their needing care as a stigma. Their concern about the effort you're making on their behalf often upsets them.

Sometimes the situation can get difficult if they challenge the kind of care you're giving and in this situation you'll be well-advised to seek help, especially if your partner refuses help. You can ask your local council for a Care Needs Assessment which may formalise arrangements and reassure your partner. If you're not sure how to start the process, begin by mentioning your concerns to your GP.

One of the things you can do in collaboration with your partner is to plan how you might adapt your home to take care of their needs. This could provide a common project and help you to bond with each other.

All of us who've ever cared for a loved one feel we could have done better. Sometimes we even blame ourselves for our shortcomings. Whatever you think, you're not a failure so never give that thought headspace. Nor should you ever feel ashamed. Guilty, maybe, but don't reverberate about it. You did your best.

Cataracts

I WANT TO TELL YOU ABOUT cataracts because it's all good news and treatment is simple. Many of us will get cataracts as we age and they can get more and more dense, restricting our eyesight. But they can be easily removed and your eyesight restored. Cataracts are small opacities in the lens of the eye so it loses its transparency and becomes cloudy. This blocks the passage of light through the eye to the retina where vision is most sharp. As the number of opacities increases with age your eyesight becomes progressively dim and vision is blurred. In severe cases the whole of the lens may be affected making the pupil look whitish in colour. As the cataracts get worse we notice we need a brighter and brighter light to read by.

And here's the good news. Your sight can be restored by a very simple and quick op. The lens can be removed by an ophthalmic surgeon and replaced by a clear artificial one. Instantly you can see clearly! The artificial lenses used by the NHS are pretty standard but you'll be astonished by the clarity of your vision which is as good as when you were a much younger person. The lens replacement operation can be done painlessly under local anaesthetic but if you'd rather, you can have a general anaesthetic. One eye is done at a time. Be prepared for your eyesight to be blurred for two to three days. Besides the standard lenses available on the NHS you can have a more sophisticated type of lens inserted into your eye which is precisely the prescription of your discarded spectacles, but at your own cost. Private surgery typically costs between £2,000-£4,000 per eye. The great thing about these lenses is you can have the lens in one eye giving you short sight for reading and the other long sight for distances. Don't worry your brain works it out in less than 24 hours.

Concentration

OUR POWERS OF CONCENTRATION ARE down to the brain and how well it's performing. A case in point... one of the classical symptoms of the menopause is an inability to concentrate. And I don't find this at all surprising as the brain has more than 80 oestrogen receptors which are keeping it in tip top condition. You can imagine what happens when that oestrogen is withdrawn and those oestrogen receptors are starved of their life blood, so to speak. Crucial brain functions like concentrating are blunted. I haven't studied the effect of testosterone on men's brains but I feel sure there are many testosterone receptors in a man's brain and if deprived of testosterone their concentration would also be lessened.

As we get older there are other important factors in play, one of the most important being blood supply. Furring up of the arteries by fat is an accompaniment to getting older. And furred up arteries can no longer deliver the amount of blood needed for all our tissues to be well-oxygenated and healthy. This applies par excellence to the brain. So loss of concentration in the older age group can be due to disease of the arteries, vascular disease. High blood pressure contributes to arterial disease and would be an additional factor. As would diabetes, both types 1 and 2, because an elevated blood sugar predisposes to furring up of the arteries.

So, living a healthy lifestyle will, as we have already discussed, help avoid these conditions which can affect concentration.

Of course, if you've had to concentrate all your life as part of your job, your concentration powers will probably remain intact longer than usual. And you can encourage your brain to concentrate with certain activities, for instance, reading, doing crosswords, playing chess, learning a new language, doing pottery or any other kind of art, playing bridge, driving, playing a sport such as golf.

And though there's little research I know of, I'm sure practising mindfulness will be good for your powers of concentration. Mindfulness involves living in the moment and therefore noticing everything around you. Mindfulness allows you to be spontaneous and spontaneity of thought and action come from somewhere deep inside your brain. I get the feeling the brain enjoys that.

Going out for a walk and practising mindfulness is an extremely good exercise in concentration for your brain. Being outside, noticing everything around you, looking at people as they pass by you, listening to bird songs, smelling flowers, watching dogs romping, looking at colours, admiring trees all involve a lot of brain activity and will help to keep your brain young and able to concentrate when you call upon it.

Cosmetic Surgery

MY PHILOSOPHY IS IF YOU want to change your appearance with cosmetic surgery, you should go ahead and do so. In my time, there's been a lot of prejudice against cosmetic surgery, being labelled vain and frivolous, but there's less stigma attached to it now. It's as well to be clear in your mind, however, why you've decided to have cosmetic surgery or you may be in for a disappointment. It won't, for instance, change your life or find you a new partner. But results are generally very good if you're in the safe hands of a skilled surgeon. I know there are people who say we should just grow old gracefully, meaning untouched by surgeons. Well, to my mind having cosmetic surgery is growing old gracefully. On the other hand, I think the obsessive pursuit of Botox and fillers is less than graceful.

How do you find a skilled surgeon? In my judgement it would be through the recommendation of a friend where you can see the best results. Beware of a cosmetic surgeon who overpromises. I'm thinking of one who guarantees the results of their work will be perfect. No good surgeon would ever promise 100% success. Also, steer clear of a surgeon who's willing to do exactly what you want without expressing their opinion on what they think you need. Run a mile from a surgeon who isn't prepared to share with you before and after pictures of their work.

Cosmetic operations of the face are probably the most common cosmetic procedure usually done to make you look younger. And they do. Nowadays, many people in their 50s upwards would like to avoid looking old as they get old. So when lines, wrinkles and bags appear, cosmetic surgery is an option.

Face lifts are the most frequent cosmetic ops. The approach for older patients is called *total facial rejuvenation* (TFR) which includes a facelift, a neck lift, eyelid repair and possibly dermabrasion, though each of these procedures can be done separately and take a much shorter time than TFR. This takes around four hours under a general anaesthetic, usually followed by a short hospital stay. After the op, your face and neck will be red and swollen and some stitches will be removed at five to seven days and the rest at two weeks. The swelling will subside in three weeks and you may feel tightness around your neck and numbness around your ears, subsiding in a few months. The results may immediately be to your liking, but that's not the end of the story. It may take up to six months to see the best effects.

Having had some cosmetic surgery (face lift) myself years ago when I was younger I would be hesitant to recommend it beyond the age of about 65. Firstly, you'd have a long general anaesthetic which isn't good as we get older. Secondly, it really is painful after the surgery and people don't tell you that. So I would ask, is it worth it? After about 65 or 70 you'll probably decide it isn't. Mind you, if you have a chronic condition like heart disease or high blood pressure you'll probably have a job finding a cosmetic surgeon who would agree to operate. Cosmetic surgery is, after all, a matter of aesthetics not health. You should also bear in mind all these procedures cost a pretty penny and the number of procedures you can have in addition to surgery has exploded. I'd recommend you go on the internet and look them up. Before you do any of this make sure you discuss it with your doctor.

In general women are opting to forgo cosmetic surgery in favour of smaller scale cosmetic treatments such as Botox and fillers which are available on the high street. I would sound a word of warning about Botox in older people as it tends to be more toxic the older we get and no one should forget Botox can have side effects. As far as fillers are concerned the older, slacker skin isn't as easy "to fill" as a younger skin so there's no guarantee where the filler will end up.

Remember "COSMETIC"

Keep in mind this advice from the GMC (General Medical Council) who oversee medical practice in the UK, when you see a cosmetic surgeon:

> **C**ONSENT – You're in charge. Your surgeon must speak to you personally and get your consent to the procedure.
> **O**PENNESS – Mistrust a doctor who isn't open and honest about their skill, experience, fees, any conflicts of interests and the risks involved.
> **S**AFETY – Check your op will take place in a safe, well-equipped hospital.
> **M**ARKETING – Your doctor must market their services responsibly and be clear about the risks involved.
> **E**XPERIENCE – Ask your doctor how many of your procedures they've done. They should have done lots, the more the better, and be able to tell you what it involves and how long it takes. Ask to see before and after pictures.
> **T**IME – Don't allow yourself to be rushed. Your doctor must give you enough time to make your decision.
> **I**NFORMATION – Your doctor must give you clear information, including details of who to contact if you're worried, and for aftercare.
> **C**OSTS – Your doctor must explain the costs clearly, including details of any fees for additional work like anaesthetics and overnight hospital stay.

Covid Boosters

I MEET QUITE A LOT OF people in my age group who've given up on Covid boosters. I absolutely haven't. As we get older and our immune system gets a little less reliable, I think it's essential that we keep stimulating it with vaccinations like flu and Covid. I know of no other way to boost the immune system. I'm particular about Covid boosters because it is such a debilitating disease. Especially now as the Covid virus is among us alongside the cold and flu viruses. We can be exposed to the Covid virus in many circumstances, without even knowing it. A friend the same age as me went to a party and three days later went down with Covid. I'm not suggesting we return to the days when we wore masks all the time in order to avoid the contagion but I feel strongly that a Covid booster is the best possible way to protect yourself from the virus. And if you do contract the virus you have a much less serious illness. To drive the point home, the friend I just mentioned who contracted Covid was better in three days, having had his Covid booster only three weeks before, which I'm pretty certain made his infection less severe. It's as well to remember that Covid can still be a nasty infection for some people especially if they haven't had all their boosters.

I have a Covid booster whenever it's offered. Being as old as I am (88) with several comorbidities such as atrial fibrillation, a lung condition dating back to my childhood when I had whooping cough, and an underactive thyroid gland, I'm in the front line to receive boosters as they become available. (Comorbidities are seen as any chronic health condition such as emphysema and liver disease.) I take advantage of boosters immediately and last time, in the spring, I had a more severe reaction to the jab than I've had previously, meaning my immune system is on good form. My arm was swollen and I couldn't raise it, my shoulder was sore, and I felt pretty lousy for two days, then I recovered. I wasn't at all worried by this reaction. In fact the opposite. I was glad my immune system was so strong it reacted strongly to the vaccine. The last time I received a Moderna vaccine which was a first for me. Previously I've always had a Pfizer vaccine and this may account for my strong reaction. It's possible the Moderna vaccine contains the variants of Covid which are now circulating and haven't been in previous vaccines. My immune system was meeting them for the first time and dealing with them, albeit in a rather dramatic but effective way.

Here are the NHS guidelines for getting the Covid-19 vaccination and the booster. If you're eligible, for example your immune system is compromised at any age, you're aged 75 and over, live in a care home you can:

- Book an appointment online or in the NHS App.
- Go to a walk-in Covid-19 vaccination site.

Some people may be able to get vaccinated at a local service, such as a community pharmacy or GP surgery, or at a care home if you live in a care home. You don't need to wait for an invitation before booking an appointment. If in doubt, ask at your local GP surgery.

I favour vaccinations because it's the only way known to science to prevent many infectious diseases, which can be serious in children.

D

Dating (Online)

ONLINE DATING IS WHERE WE'RE at. People looking for friendship, companionship, and even long-term relationships go online these days to find that special person. In our shorthand world, people are looking to build connections, find friends, even find love. It's claimed for one of the most well-known dating sites that every 14 minutes someone finds love. At the very least, many people going online hope they'll find a partner who will share interests and to whom they can get close. And sometimes a dating site is just plain useful because it may put you in contact with singles who live near you and you have the connection of proximity.

I've never used a dating app myself and I doubt I ever shall. Why? Well, when I was younger and working for a pharmaceutical company, I did a great deal of travelling and cultivated an aura of not being available, not approachable. "Please don't speak to me" was the vibe I gave off. I think I feel the same now. So being confronted with someone I don't know I would probably start wearing my old armour.

I confess to preferring to meet anyone face to face but I guess that's what comes on the first date. I want to make eye contact, I want to read body language, see faces, see responses. What makes them laugh? What makes them shocked? And find out first-hand what their expectations are, if any, of this meeting? What about their family? And hobbies, outside interests and travelling? Do you feel any chemistry? Do you feel there's enough in common for a friendship? A long relationship? Do you feel that you'd be happy going away with this person, and sharing a room? And almost certainly in this situation, how would you feel about sex with them?

The expectations of online dating vary quite a lot from what previous generations were looking for. Nowadays, quite a lot of people go online in order to meet a sexual partner. And if you choose to go online, you should expect this, even though it may not chime with you. I have a 70-year-old friend who met a man online also in his 70s. They got on well, she enjoyed his company. He cooked her a lovely meal and she felt flattered by his attention. It turned out he expected sex after his cheffing duties. Initially she enjoyed that, but was knocked off her feet when he confessed openly that he was ethically non-monogamous (!) and he met many women and had sex with them. He was not looking for an exclusive relationship and she was. Consternation. There was not the marriage of minds and expectations.

Having said all that, many people do meet people they really like, form a long-term relationship and marry, living happily ever after. So if you feel you'd like to take the plunge and try your luck with online dating don't hesitate. Just do it! But look after yourself.

Staying safe

Online dating can be fun and exciting and most people are genuine, but you have to be savvy to avoid disappointment or worse, being catfished. Here are a few things to bear in mind.

- Keep the conversation within the app and don't share your phone number until you're comfortable meeting.

- Don't let them pressure you to do something you don't want to.
- Don't share any nude pictures!
- Don't share too much personal information and definitely don't share financial information online.
- Never send money!
- If they're too good to be true, they probably are. Do a "Google image search" of the person's photo and if it comes back as a stock photo or photo of someone else, report them (see instructions at the end).
- If their answers are just one word, repetitive or don't make sense they could be a bot and not a real person. Report and delete them immediately.
- Before meeting, screenshot their photos and your conversations in case the date turns bad.
- Always tell someone where and what time your date is and check in with them after.

How do I verify the authenticity of a photograph?

If a picture seems too perfect it could have been created by AI so if you're unsure that you're talking to the person in the pictures use Google image search to check for authenticity. Here's how:

1. Take a screenshot of the photo on your phone.
2. Go to Google.com and click on the camera icon in the search bar (next to the microphone image).
3. Your picture gallery will open up – tap the picture you want to search.

If Google finds an exact match, check the website where the photo appears. If you find the picture is their profile photo on their social media or on their personal website, it's likely they're who they claim to be. However, if you find their picture (possibly with a different name) in an online catalogue or in a stock image library, stay away. They're most probably not who they say they are.

Dementia/Alzheimer's

I CARED FOR MY HUSBAND WITH dementia for three years so I understand how difficult it is for someone to look after a person with dementia and how it can completely take over your life. As the dementia gets worse, the stresses and strains imposed on you increase almost daily and it's exhausting. Few people can appreciate the strain you're under, not even family, and you may find yourself shouldering the whole burden of daily care on your own. As someone who's been in your place I would advise you never to do that, but to seek help as soon as you suspect your partner has early dementia. Seek help from your doctor and from family members who can help you personally on a day-to-day basis. I'm sympathetic to people who feel no one else understands what they're going through because, frankly, no one else does understand other than someone who's done it.

In the early stages it's hard to know if someone really does have dementia because the changes may be subtle, but the symptoms of Alzheimer's will gradually appear and worsen – loss of short-term memory, looking endlessly for a purse or a wallet, not paying bills, not preparing meals, not remembering appointments, getting lost travelling outside of the familiar local neighbourhood, being bewildered by anything new – people, places and things, and being unable to make a decision.

More and more families are worrying that a parent or relative is in the early stages of dementia.

So how will you know if it's Alzheimer's?

People with Alzheimer's tend to become more and more withdrawn, losing interest in life and what's going on around them. They're often sad, anxious, frightened and get upset easily.

Doctors have a test, a series of simple questions, they use to assess if a person has dementia. These questions test memory, their sense of time and place and perception of who and where they are. I've extracted a few to give you some background to the test.

> How old are you?
> Which day of the week is it?
> Which month are we in?
> Can you remember the year?
> What's your address?
> What town do you live in?
> Can you remember which school you went to?
> And what about the date of World War I/World War II?
> What's the name of our Prime Minister?
> Who's on the throne at the moment?
> Can you say the months of the year backwards?
> Can you count from 1 to 20?
> Can you count from 20 to 1?

The number of questions that the person can't answer will contribute to a diagnosis of dementia.

You might like to look at the helpful information on the Alzheimer's Society's website www.alzheimers.org.uk.

How common is Alzheimer's?

I recall, as a junior doctor more than 50 years ago, Alzheimer's and dementia were relatively uncommon but over the ensuing years they've been diagnosed more and more frequently. This is partly because we're better at diagnosing dementia, but it's also because we're living longer. In the main, dementia comes on in the latter part of life in the 60s, 70s and 80s and many more people are living longer than they did when I was a junior doctor.

Some stats are revealing. Currently nearly a million people are living with dementia in the UK and this is projected to rise to 1.4 million by 2040[10]. But we also know that many more people living with the early signs of Alzheimer's are still undiagnosed. The same goes for the rest of the world where over 55 million people were living with dementia in 2020. This number will almost double every 20 years, reaching 78 million in 2030 and 139 million in 2050.[11]

If you feel your memory is failing there are remedies. You can try giving it a boost and you may lower the possibility of developing dementia. Given the right stimulation we now know the brain can repair itself by growing new brain cells. And the stimulation the brain needs is exercise, thinking. This very simple expedient helps the brain to renew itself by releasing hormones that stimulate not only brain cells to grow but also brain connections. The upshot is that every time you think for example reading a book, learning a new language, performing a difficult task, you're keeping your brain young and your memory fresh. Here are some tricks to put your memory through its paces every day. I use the "grid" all the time.

Keeping your memory sharp

- When you lose something, remember it's always where you left it and you can find it in the "grid". This is a map you make in your head or on paper of everything you've done since you last had the object and where you've been. Write down the last six

---

10   https://www.alzheimers.org.uk
11   https://www.alzint.org/

things you did prior to losing it and where you were for each one. If necessary, draw a grid on a piece of paper of the last five/six things you were doing down one side, and where you were along the bottom. Then complete the grid. The lost article is in one of the squares you've drawn. All you have to do to find what you've lost is to "look" in each square.

- When we try to remember several things, use a mnemonic. When I was a medical student there was so much to remember, we had mnemonics for everything. One of my favourites was a mnemonic to remember the cranial nerves (12 of them) which are Olfactory, Optic, Oculomotor, Trochlear, Trigeminal, Facial, Abducens, Vestibulocochlear, Glossopharyngeal, Vagus, Accessory and Hypoglossal. The mnemonic we had is really rather scandalous and it had been thought up by the boys. Of course. The mnemonic that I remember everybody saying was, "Oh, Oh, Oh, To Try Feeling A Vivacious Girl's Vagina, All, Hot." So, for example, when you have several tasks to remember, tasks such as going to the chemist, putting away your underwear and phoning a friend you can fit them into one easy to remember word. By assembling the first letters of each task you have CUP (chemist/underwear/phone) and it will keep your memory sharp.
- Don't we all walk into a room and then forget why we're there. My routine is to go back to where I came from, look around for some clue to jog my memory about what I need and I don't leave until I've remembered the reason. Then I repeat it to myself while I'm trying to find it.
- After reading a book or watching a film, write down a summary or do one in your head, in chronological order, including the names of characters.
- When doing a weekly shop find as many items as you can without referring to your shopping list.

So what causes dementia?

The root cause of dementia is the destruction of brain cells preventing connections passing messages from one part of the brain to another or from one cell to another. So far we've tracked down two possible culprits, amyloid and tau, both proteins. Normally they exist inside nerve cells but in Alzheimer's they leak out, forming tangles and plaques around and between brain cells. These tangles are toxic enough to kill off brain cells and disrupt pathways that keep brain cells connected to each other.

The hippocampus is one of the first parts of the brain affected by this disruption. It's responsible for memory and learning so the early signs of Alzheimer's are often memory failure and difficulty learning.

What does the future look like?

At the present time there is no cure for dementia, but there are drugs that can slow down its progress. These drugs, aspirin, NSAIDs and possibly HRT, will protect against worsening of Alzheimer's, slow its progress and help you retain your memory, keep you emotionally stable, able to concentrate, assess new information and make decisions.

Two of the latest drugs for Alzheimer's are Leqembi and Kisunla. They are called "disease modifying drugs" (DMD) because they target amyloid plaques, and in the early stage of Alzheimer's may slow down the progress of dementia.

The development of anti-tau vaccines are already in clinical trials giving hope for the future.

Diet for dementia..?

Is there a dementia diet? Not that I know of but there are some foods that help to keep your brain healthy. Make sure you eat them once or twice a week.

- Vitamin-rich foods. The brain gobbles up B vitamins particularly B12 so feed your brain with fish, eggs, yoghurt, shellfish, dairy, fortified cereals, chicken and red meat, enough to cover the palm of your hand. Remember vegetables don't contain vitamin B12 as it's an animal derived vitamin.
- Omega-3s. Fill up your body with omega-3s by eating nuts and seeds, fatty fish (salmon, mackerel, herring), shellfish, soya beans, flaxseed oil, some fruits (kiwi, papaya, oranges and berries) and avocados.
- Couple of squares of dark chocolate a day.
- Lots of fruits, veg, pulses, beans, dark green leaves and tomatoes.
- No cigarettes or vapes, and very little alcohol.

So does memory loss automatically mean dementia?

Absolutely not! From the age of 50 we can spot lapses of memory. The first one is nearly always being unable to remember names. That can creep on to where you left your keys, remembering to turn off the lights and keeping appointments.

You might describe this as "benign" loss of memory because it's not the more serious memory loss of dementia which is wider and deeper. That stems from losing the ability to concentrate or to make decisions.

Furthermore it's impossible to cure. So someone has to look for their purse or wallet over and over again. Deep memory loss leads to forgetting how to drive a car, forgetting your address, and forgetting where the post office is.

Dr Miriam Stoppard

Depression

MOST OF US GET DEPRESSED at times. I know I do. Dealing with the ups and downs of everyday life such as a friend letting us down, losing a job, a rift in the family, the news that you've got cancer, someone close to you dying, can knock us for six. This, I personally would define as having a depressed mood, feeling low, feeling blue, so this kind of depression is about feelings and we can usually snap out of it. We're all familiar with depression as a mood, so we talk about "Monday morning blues" and the "baby blues" after having a child. These negative feelings may combine to make us feel down in the dumps, apprehensive, gloomy, miserable, low, lifeless, flat, feel fed up and cheesed off with life.

But this isn't *clinical depression*. Clinical depression is deep and unremitting, combining low energy, a sense of being down in spirits, with feeling worthless, and having a sense of hopelessness and uselessness. Don't wait. Consult your doctor as early as you can because when depression takes hold, it becomes more difficult to treat.

It could be at certain stages of our lives we become more vulnerable to depression. Getting older would be one (more than 6 in 10 people in the UK aged 65+ have had depression and anxiety[12] and nearly 1 in 10 aged 75+ deal with depression[13]), having to face retirement and beyond would be another. Having lost self-confidence in our middle years – the menopause for women, a midlife

---

12   https://www.england.nhs.uk/2020/01/older-people-encouraged-to-ditch-stiff-upper-lip-approach-to-mental-ill-health/
13   https://sphr.nihr.ac.uk/news-and-events/more-older-people-with-depression-could-benefit-from-non-drug-treatments/

crisis for men – we get the feeling we're lagging behind. As we get older it's not just a feeling, we start to *know* we're lagging behind: we can't dance the way we used to, we can't play tennis the way we used to, we can't go for a jog the way we used to, and we can't have sex the way we used to. The answer is, if we can manage it, to accept there are now constraints on what our bodies are capable of and to celebrate what we still can do, rather than concentrating on what we can't. Depression is by no means inevitable at this stage of life and it's usually people who have suffered trauma in childhood or feel life has treated them unfairly who are likely to get depressed in later life.

Deep, prolonged clinical depression is serious. It slows down both body and mind. A depressed person can't think properly because thought is slowed down too. Even our internal organs slow down, the bowels slow down so that constipation is quite common in depressed people. Depression is often worse first thing in the morning and improves as the day goes on. A depressed person may blame themselves for things going wrong so they feel guilty and full of self-reproach. Rarely they'll feel so helpless, so ashamed and so guilt-ridden that suicide seems the only way out.

Trying to feel better

Try to be proactive when you're feeling unhappy

Work helps you to forget and stops brooding so increase your workload and keep to as normal a routine as you can. Doing a geographic to change your environment such as going away for a holiday, will give you a new point of view to help resolve conflicts that may be precipitating your crisis. Any activity helps to reduce sadness.

Finishing something brings a sense of achievement and self-worth which is an antidote to depression. This reminds me of when

I came home from school and found my mum on her knees scrubbing the kitchen floor. I knew she was trying to cope with unhappiness.

Ask for help

Please don't hesitate to lean on people. Get help dealing with the problems of everyday life. Join a self-help group. Don't be afraid to approach groups such as the Samaritans. Try helping other people and if you ever contemplate suicide, talk to someone right away. Avoid being alone and, where you can, surround yourself with cheerful people.

Don't wait

Depression can recur, so at the first sign of worsening mood get in touch with someone who knows your mental history, before your daily life is affected.

Sex

Good wholesome sex makes all aspects of life brighter, so if your libido isn't low, speak to your partner about relishing mutual enjoyment of your sex life.

Some thoughts on recovering from depression

I'd like you to know about some strategies that could help you rebuild your self-confidence and regain control of your life while you're recovering from depression.

- Make a list of things that you have to do each day, beginning with the most important and tick the boxes as you go.
- Tackle one task at a time, and reflect on what you have achieved when each is done.

- Pat yourself on the back each time. Say to yourself, 'Well done!'
- Set aside a few minutes each day to relax by breathing deeply or stretching.
- Exercise regularly to help manage feelings of stress.
- Eat a healthy diet.
- Take up a pastime or hobby that distracts you from worries.
- Join a support group where you can meet other people who have had similar experiences.
- Plan a few "rewards" for putting in the effort – meet a friend for coffee, go to the cinema, buy yourself a new lipstick, get some new jeans or a new dress, buy the sunglasses you've always wanted.

These days, there are several ways in which a depressed person can start feeling normal again without the use of drugs like antidepressants. Psychological treatments are valuable because they bring together your mind and your feelings.

All of these psychological treatments work. Personally, I really believe in psychodrama. I made a TV documentary in Seattle, US where abused girls and women acted out their abuse, some using a 4ft penis to explore their deepest darkest feelings. It was harrowing, but it worked dramatically.

Psychodrama helps you act out feelings of being depressed and the circumstances which have led you to be depressed. Experiences are recreated and you get in touch with feelings that are locked inside of you and make your feelings work for you. One of the most important aspects of psychodrama and psychotherapy is sharing your depression with others in a group. By sharing theirs with you and vice versa, healing begins.

Counselling will help you by examining your problems with a counsellor who finds out the facts to separate reality from fantasy. Together with the counsellor you make a plan of action giving emotional support while difficult decisions are being made and acted upon.

Psychotherapy is a special form of counselling that enables new emotional learning by exploring inner conflicts causing your depression with your therapist so you can cope better with your feelings.

The Importance of Exercise

I have only one helpful hint to give you and that's exercise, exercise, exercise. The benefits are legion. When I was researching my book on healthy ageing I came up with more than 30. Nothing benefits from exercise like your brain. Your brain loves it and here are a few stats to prove it.

The MHAW[14] report gives us a good idea of how exercise boosts our mental health.

Regular physical activity is important for overall physical health	84% agreed
Regular physical activity is important for mental health and wellbeing	82% agreed
Physical activity contributes to better quality sleep	80% agreed
Being physically active can reduce the risk of depression	76% agreed
Physical activity can help me to manage stress	74% agreed
I feel more energised and alert after being physically active	73% agreed
Physical activity improves mood	71% agreed

---

14   MHF - MHAW Movement - Report 2024

I feel more confident and positive about myself when I engage in physical activity	70% agreed

Self Affirmations

When I was going through a bad patch in my 50s due to business worries, self-affirmations were a life saver. I had them on post-its all over the house so I couldn't escape these positive images of myself. They could help you too. Constantly undermining yourself can arise from bad experiences in childhood at school and at teen age, that have remained unresolved. The longer you've been grappling with them the more difficult they are to erase. The "self-talk" of positive affirmations can do much to unpick negative self-image. They also make you think of yourself differently so you boost self-confidence and self-esteem. I'm sure you can come up with your own affirmations. I include some I'm helped by. By all means say them to yourself silently but saying them out loud is much more powerful. Your own voice can teach you to feel good about yourself.

- I'm a good person.
- I believe in my potential to succeed.
- I can make my life better and better.
- I love and accept myself for who I am.
- I wasn't put on earth just to please others.
- I'm getting stronger, healthier and more energetic.
- I deserve to be happy.

Repeat this list once a day and whenever you're feeling low.

Antidepressants

In addition to psychotherapy, you and your doctor could consider antidepressants which come with different active ingredients, all aimed at improving our mood.

Even though antidepressants are a key part of treating depression in young adults, opinions vary on how effective they are in relieving symptoms in older people. When they do work, they work very well but they work better in some situations than in others. Furthermore, they shouldn't be used for the treatment of mild forms of depression. It's moderate and serious depression they're intended for. Bear in mind they also have side effects depending on the type you take, so you should discuss the pros and cons with your doctor before starting on them.

The main aim of antidepressants is to make depression better and prevent it coming back. You can expect to feel emotionally stable again and get relief from restlessness, anxiety and sleep problems. They also prevent suicidal thoughts.

What antidepressants are available?

We have several to suit different people.
- Tricyclic antidepressants (TCAs)
- Selective serotonin reuptake inhibitors (SSRIs)
- Selective serotonin noradrenaline reuptake inhibitors (SNRIs)

They're all effective and can take up to three weeks before you feel the full effect. You and your doctor have to work together to find one that suits you, and so you may have to ring the changes in order to be satisfied and happy with your medication. Antidepressants work on chemical messengers in the brain which pass on signals to other parts, called neurotransmitters. Neurotransmitters you may have heard of are serotonin and dopamine.

Not everyone agrees with the use of antidepressants in old age as even the gentlest ones (SSRIs, mirtazapine) can cause side effects like headaches, dry mouth, weight gain and feeling sleepy, in fact mirtazapine is excellent for treating sleep disturbances in older people. At the moment SSRIs are the most commonly prescribed antidepressant for older people and for those with dementia. By the way, please don't feel any shame about needing an antidepressant. I see them as an essential vitamin needed to get through a difficult time and may be needed in the long term.

You'll need to take your antidepressant every day, usually starting at a low dose and increasing. The goal in the first months is to relieve your negative feelings and where possible free you from depression completely. Once this has been achieved, the treatment continues for at least six to 12 months and then your doctor may be prepared to wean you off medication by lowering the dose over eight to 12 weeks.

You may temporarily have sleep problems, nausea and restlessness while coming off an antidepressant. Never, never, never try to stop your antidepressant quickly.

Side effects

Bear in mind, like all medications, antidepressants can have side effects and over half of people who take antidepressants get them, usually in the first three weeks of treatment. You may have a dry mouth, headaches, dizziness, restlessness and sexual problems depending on which drug you take and the dose. Remember an antidepressant may make the side effects of other drugs worse. This kind of drug interaction is more common in older people and people with chronic illnesses who are taking several different medicines. Particularly important in older people is the fact that antidepressants can cause dizziness and unsteadiness, increasing the risk of falls and fractures.

Dr Miriam Stoppard

Divorce

DIVORCE CAN BE MORE DIFFICULT as we get older than when we were younger. For one thing, you may not have the stamina you had then and divorce takes stamina. For another, you may not have the emotional resilience and some divorces demand great staying power. According to government stats between 2005 and 2015 the number of men divorcing aged 65 and over went up by 23% and the number of women of the same age divorce increased by 38%. Divorces were first granted in civil partnerships in 2007. Between 2007 and 2015, only 131 men and women aged 65 and over ended a civil partnership in England and Wales making up 1.1% of all divorces[15].

While some people see divorce as liberation and a new, exciting phase of their lives, others may feel they've been left on the shelf, that they're no longer attractive, and they'll have difficulty ever finding someone who wants to strike up a relationship with them. After living so long with a partner, it may be difficult to contemplate living alone. It's especially hard for women who've been left for a younger model.

Other divorce stats show around 80,000 divorces were granted in England and Wales in 2022, and in 2021, 1 in 4 took place after the age of 50[16].

Retirement provides opportunities to explore hobbies, to travel, to meet new people and it's common for couples to drift apart as a result of their newfound freedom. New laws have made the

---

15   https://www.ons.gov.uk/peoplepopulationandcommunity/birthsdeath-sandmarriages/marriagecohabitationandcivilpartnerships/articles/marriageand-divorceontheriseat65andover/2017-07-18
16   https://www.legalandgeneral.com/articles/enjoying-retirement/reasons-for-divorce-in-retirement/

divorce process simpler. In April 2022, the UK government allowed couples to choose the option of a 'no-fault divorce', meaning they no longer need to lay blame to part ways.

An increase in divorces for opposite-sex couples could be down to wives being more financially independent. Whereas women were once tied forever to their other halves due to having no means of managing alone, that's no longer the case. Deciding to separate is easier once children have grown up and settled down with families of their own and, although the sudden break-up of older parents can be a shock to their children and grandchildren, it's easier than divorcing when the kids are still living at home.

Could the increase in older people forming new relationships be due to living longer? Fifty years ago, an average man could expect to live to 69 and a woman to 74. Today, a man aged 55 has an average life expectancy of 84, and a 1 in 4 chance he'll live to 92. For a woman of the same age, the average life expectancy is 87, with a 1 in 4 chance of living to 94 and a 1 in 10 chance of living to 98. For these reasons, divorces are more common now, and there are more people in the marriage market.

The consequences of divorce can vary enormously. For a woman who hasn't got a career to go back to and feels too old to start a new one, it's perfectly reasonable to feel, having brought up a family and helping a man to achieve success in his career, that she deserves financial compensation. A divorcee who's anxious about her finances and in particular, alimony, may fight hard for her dues. This hurt and anxiety may make a woman feel that her divorce signals the end of her life, pretty much. There may also be the disruption and sense of loss of security of having to sell a family home.

On the other hand many women find that life is better after divorce. Vistas open up, a new job, voluntary work – always good for the morale – and taking up new interests, especially those that she's longed to do all her life, can feel like a new lease of life. If dating is on the agenda a woman who's led a rather boring sex life with her partner can discover a whole new kind of sexuality she was unaware of before. Contrary to what you thought, you may not have a low sex drive and find post-divorce sex has opened up new ways to enjoy it. You may even feel reborn. Don't forget you're in the prime of your life and, with a fair wind, you have quite a few more years left. You've been through the menopause so you need have no worries about getting pregnant.

Men by and large see divorce differently from women, and it may be the domestic side of life that affects them most. After all, they've always had a partner to look after them, to get breakfast, cook meals, do the laundry and make the home comfortable for them. Problem is with newfound earning power, more women leave men than men leave women. Men tend to stay put in a marriage because they have quite a cushy life. If a confident, self-assertive woman decides to get out of a marriage, the man understandably feels abandoned, even depressed. This may trigger him to start looking to re-establish his old way of life and seek a lasting relationship with a new wife. The truth is, marriage may be better suited to men than women. There are plenty of statistics to show that men are happiest, the least depressed, and in the best health when they're married. The result is they seek re-marriage quite quickly after divorce.

Divorce in retirement

Don't make a rushed decision

A divorce is a life-changing event so you have to make sure you and your partner have taken everything into account before going through with it. Take time to sit down and talk about it in great detail.

Tell the children together
Telling your children is difficult whether they're still young or adults with their own family. You and your partner should tell them together and prepare for questions they might ask.

It's your decision, no one else's
By all means talk to family and friends about wanting a divorce but don't necessarily be influenced by what they say. Pursue your own agenda.

Don't hesitate to seek help
Going through a divorce is a stressful time so if you feel you can't cope, make an appointment with a therapist who can help you through it.

Talk finances
If you have been married for a long time you probably have joint assets that need to be divided. Talk with your partner about how you might do this and see a financial advisor if you need to.

Don't talk about your divorce on social media
It's quite common for people to overshare their private life on social media but try to refrain from it as it would only invite criticism not support.

Driving

IN THE LAST FEW YEARS, I've been asked several times to go on morning television to debate the age I think a driving licence should no longer be issued. But I believe the ability to drive safely is down to the individual and therefore it's not tenable to stipulate an age limit. At 88 I have just stopped driving – although not because I wanted to but because it was the safe thing to do.

I've always loved cars. So much so that as a junior doctor I became the medical officer at the Castle Combe race track in Wiltshire where I would drag injured young men out of wrecked cars. I've always particularly loved fast cars, owning three Porsches over the years. But I had to give those up in my early 60s when the car's reflexes seemed to be faster than mine. And I think it's worth expanding here on my experience driving to Toulouse airport which I mentioned in the section on "Balance and Unsteadiness" because it has an important message on road safety. So after driving along a motorway in the south of France to Toulouse airport on my journey home to London, in airport security I suddenly found I couldn't move. The room was spinning and I was being sick. I was taken to A&E and after that to a French hospital for investigation.

The incident in airport security was nasty but that isn't the point. The point is 20 minutes earlier I'd been on a motorway and if I'd had this attack of vertigo while driving I would have endangered the lives of others, and my own. As a result, my sons said, "Sorry Mum, no more driving." And they were right. I've accepted it. So while we may feel at a ripe old age, we're still fit to drive and want to go on driving, there are other considerations we should be mindful of.

In France there's no age limit to when you can hold a driving licence nor is there one in the UK but from the age of 70 you have to renew your licence every three years. As long as you can see clearly enough and you're able enough there's no real reason for you not to have a driving licence. Except as we get older, night vision becomes dim and misty. Night driving should be a no no as soon as your vision deteriorates, and your reflexes slow down.

If we're strictly honest with ourselves we know when we reach the point where we should give up driving, despite curtailing our freedom of movement which is so precious. If you're not sure the moment has come, try asking one of the younger generation. It was my sons who questioned my ability to continue driving and who persuaded me to give it up. I just had to face up to it. I feel my wings have been clipped but with the slowing of my reflexes I know in my heart I shouldn't drive any more. Don't let this make you feel excluded. You needn't be. There's always public transport and a younger friend who may offer to drive you and apps such as Uber have brought down the cost of taxi journeys considerably. It may also be far cheaper to travel everywhere by taxi than to face the increased costs of insurance in older age along with road tax and petrol.

Drugs/Medications

YOU'D BE VERY LUCKY INDEED if you reached your 60s and weren't taking one medication or another to treat a long-term ailment. In older age we lean heavily on a variety of drugs to keep our bodies ticking over. Always remember that taking medication doesn't mean you're a lesser person for doing so. In fact, quite the opposite. The drugs we need at the end of our lives are the ones that keep us healthy, seeing out our old age. So we should be grateful for them.

As the body gets older, however, it doesn't handle drugs the way it did when it was younger. In the first place, drugs tend to stay longer in the body than they used to, and this is largely because they take longer to exit the stomach and the intestine. This results in some drugs having a longer duration of action and possibly more side effects.

When I take medication, I try to help the body use it efficiently. First thing I do is to drink a lot of water and this isn't just to help the drugs slide down easily. The stomach responds to water by making acid and most drugs are more easily broken down and more efficiently absorbed if the stomach contents are acid. So whenever I take medicines, I drink three of glasses of water, one to take the medicine down and the second and third to make sure they've reached my stomach. As the ageing body contains less water than it used to, a couple of glasses with your medicines will also help to keep your body hydrated.

As we get older and our mouths are drier, swallowing tablets can be difficult, so here's a way to make it easier. I place the tablet on my tongue and then I take a sip of water but don't swallow. I drop my chin towards my chest and then swallow. What you mustn't do is to throw your head backwards in an effort to get the pill down because our swallowing mechanism in this position is very inefficient and the tablet may get stuck. I also put off my morning coffee for half an hour as caffeine slows down the absorption of the l-thyroxine I take for my underactive thyroid.

These days, we're fortunate to have a myriad drugs to treat almost anything. But I'm going to concentrate on what I would call "life-saving everyday meds" that quite a few of us need to ensure our health and longevity. The drugs I'm referring to would be statins, anticoagulants, beta-blockers, vitamin D and also some drugs used prophylactically like vaginal oestrogen to prevent UTIs (urinary tract infections) and the latest treatments for dementia. I'll also mention weight loss drugs.

Statins are used to lower cholesterol and so protect against heart attacks. I've been a keen advocate of them ever since they were first discovered. Anticoagulants would be used if you have a condition such as AF (atrial fibrillation), to stop the blood from clotting inside your heart. We use beta-blockers to keep the heart beating regularly and diuretics as first-line treatment for high blood pressure; vitamin D is essential to keep bones strong and resist fractures; intravaginal oestrogen is especially useful in chronic urinary tract infections to ensure the bladder and the urethra (the tube leading from the bladder to the outside) are healthy and able to resist infections.

Statins

So how did I get started on statins when I was relatively young in my late 50s? I was arriving in San Francisco for a medical conference and in a taxi going to my hotel when I had an attack of excruciating chest pain, pain I'd never felt before. I thought to myself, this is either a heart attack or I've got a stomach ulcer. I decided I could distinguish between these two conditions by taking an antacid medicine to relieve my stomach pain so I asked the driver to pull over at the next pharmacy. It was about 4am by this time – and I got some Pepto Bismol which I glugged down and waited to see if it would relieve my pain. It did. I'd excluded the possibility of an acute heart condition. It turned out I had a stomach ulcer.

Nevertheless, when I got back to the UK, I went to see a cardiologist to assess my cardiac function. My heart was declared okay but he suggested that I take statins in order to prevent heart disease in the future. I went on statins as a preventative. Statins can vary in dose and usually your doctor will start you on a low dose and raise it if necessary to keep your cholesterol levels as near normal as possible.

When statins first appeared there were some doctors who thought they shouldn't be taken universally. One of the reasons was great emphasis was placed on a rather rare side effect, muscle pain. Statins came back in favour when it was shown that muscle pain due to statins was uncommon. Nowadays the majority of doctors see the necessity for statins in older people, both as a treatment to lower cholesterol and as a preventive to stop cholesterol rising. At the present time more than seven million Brits take statins to keep their cholesterol normal. In a recent study of treatment for CLL (chronic lymphocytic leukaemia), the most common form of blood cancer in adults in the UK, plus a similar condition called SSL (small lymphocytic lymphoma) out of the 1,467 involved, about 420 were taking statins and five years on they were 61% less likely to have died from the cancers than others. Their original cancer was 26% less likely to have progressed. Is this a whole new era for statins[17]?

Anticoagulants

These have become a mainstay for treating cardiac and vascular problems. An anticoagulant is a blood thinner and stops the blood from clotting. It can also dissolve clots.

When you're started on anticoagulant treatment you may get injections such as warfarin and then once your blood has stabilised you may go onto a tablet, which is what I take, one a day. If you have a blockage in any main artery you may be given an anticoagulant, probably an injectable one at first, superseded a week or so later by a tablet you take daily.

I'm on one such drug because I have AF, atrial fibrillation, where the heart beats irregularly. Small clots tend to form in the heart with AF and can be treated with an anticoagulant tablet to dissolve them so they don't get into the general circulation, something that has to be prevented because a clot might travel to the brain and cause a stroke. Taking an oral anticoagulant couldn't be simpler as no check-up tests are necessary. I was put on a beta-blocker as a protection against having repeated attacks of AF. It just steadies my heart and stops it from beating too fast or beating irregularly.

---

17 https://b-s-h.org.uk/about-us/news/statin-linked-to-blood-cancer-survival#:~:text=Thursday%2C%201%20May%202025,the%20risk%20of%20disease%20progression

Oestrogen

Yes, I bet if you're an older woman you thought you were far too old for HRT. But there's a condition where older women are greatly helped by using a special form of it, to treat and prevent chronic urinary tract infections (UTIs). Like many women my age, I get UTIs, and if you've ever had one, you know how debilitating the pain can be and how ill it makes you feel. Your inflamed bladder wants to empty all the time so you have to go to the loo every few minutes.

Repeat urinary tract infections are also bad for your kidneys and liver, so it's worth trying everything to prevent them. It's not an easy job because if repeated courses of antibiotics have been used, your infection may be resistant to some antibiotics. Your doctor will have to search for one to which you are sensitive with urine tests.

Since I turned 80, I've had several UTIs which ruled my life while I was having them and I resented it. So I decided to tackle the infections in a different way. The truth is, along with the rest of body tissues, the lining of the bladder and the urethra, the tube which connects the bladder to the outside and the lining of the vagina, become thin, dry and vulnerable to infections. Could I restore their health?

Well, it's possible to do this by giving them a healthy dose of oestrogen via the vagina. Using an intravaginal cream or pessary, the oestrogen seeps through the tissues to the bladder and the urethra, returning them to a more youthful state and able to resist infections. Don't worry, intravaginal oestrogen is safe because it goes no further than your pelvis and doesn't affect the rest of your body. I strongly believe in vaginal oestrogen for UTIs and if you're a woman who suffers from them, I would recommend asking your doctor for a trial run, and use the cream or a pessary twice a week.

Since I started on intravaginal oestrogen I haven't had a urinary tract infection[18].

Polypill

You'd think because there are several drugs aimed at protecting and supporting the heart, they might be grouped together in one tablet, wouldn't you? Well, you'd be right. There is a polypill containing a statin, a diuretic to control high blood pressure and a small dose of aspirin to thin the blood. Advocates of the polypill say it could prevent hundreds of thousands of heart attacks and strokes. But this preventive medicine, even in its latest version, hasn't been taken up with any enthusiasm by the NHS, possibly because of cost, as there are three drugs in one pill. A newer polypill with two ingredients is now available. You could speak to your doctor if you are interested in trying it.

Beta blockers

Beta blockers are possibly best known for helping actors get over stage fright. They don't actually relieve the actors' anxiety, what they do is to relieve some of the symptoms of anxiety like palpitations and over-breathing. Beta blockers belong to a group of drugs used mainly to manage abnormal heart rhythms and keep the heart beating regularly. I take one myself for AF, atrial fibrillation, where the heart beats irregularly and there's a danger of clots forming inside the heart. They may then find their way into the general circulation and cause damage such as stroke when they get into the smaller arteries of the brain and block them. Beta blockers are also prescribed to treat angina, heart pain which comes on with effort, and to lower blood pressure. People who've had a heart

---

18   https://pmc.ncbi.nlm.nih.gov/articles/PMC3878051/
https://pubmed.ncbi.nlm.nih.gov/37178856/

attack, have valve disease of the heart or are in heart failure may be prescribed beta blockers too.

Watch out for side effects like tiredness which I had myself when I started on beta blockers. I felt I couldn't drag one foot after the other. I told my doctor and the dose was halved. My tiredness disappeared. Other common side effects are feeling dizzy and light-headed. Your toes and fingers may feel cold because as your blood pressure is lower it's difficult for blood to reach your extremities. For the same reason men may have difficulty achieving and maintaining an erection as the heart beats with less force than before. If you're put on a beta blocker avoid caffeine, antihistamines, cold cures and alcohol, all of which lower the effect of beta blockers. Also try to limit your intake of potassium-rich foods like bananas, papayas, tomatoes, avocados and kale. To combat tiredness keep hydrated and keep moving about to boost your energy levels.

Dry Eyes, Dry Mouth

AS WE GET OLDER, OUR bodies slow down and one of the effects is fewer tears and less saliva, so your eyes can feel sore and prickly and your mouth is often dry. Dry eyes are due to the tear glands (lachrymal) failing to work properly to produce enough tears to keep the eyes well lubricated. A dry mouth is caused by a shortage of saliva as the salivary glands produce less. Both of these conditions are easy to alleviate. I would suggest you ask your local pharmacist for advice. They can give you artificial tears for the eyes, which you should use several times a day and definitely before sleeping. Artificial saliva will relieve your dry mouth. I suffer with a dry mouth myself, and I find it's almost totally relieved by chewing gum, though that's not a very attractive habit.

There's one condition where both the eyes and mouth are dry. This is Sjögren's syndrome (SS) where there's also arthritis of the hands and feet, resembling rheumatoid arthritis. This is a condition where the membranes inside the joints, the salivary glands and the lacrimal glands tend to dry out. SS shows up in a blood test. You should see a specialist for a treatment plan including oral steroids, possibly in the long-term.

Here are some more things you can do to help ease the symptoms of Sjögren's syndrome, recommended by the NHS[19].

Do

- Sip water all day.
- Look after mouth hygiene by brushing your teeth two or three times a day using fluoride toothpaste, chewing sugar-free gum and having dental check-ups every six months.
- Moist air helps your symptoms so use a humidifier and put plants in your home to increase water vapour in the air.
- To help stop your eyes drying out when you're outdoors wear sunglasses with enclosed sides.
- See your optician regularly for eye checks.
- Eat a healthy, balanced diet – in particular, include foods rich in omega-3, such as oily fish and walnuts.
- SS can cause muscle and joint pain so take painkillers such as paracetamol and see your doctor if you need something stronger.
- You may have vaginal dryness so use a vaginal moisturiser and a pH controlled water-based lubricant during sex. If you'd like to try intravaginal oestrogen speak to your doctor.
- Use emollients to cleanse your skin because soap makes your skin dry.

---

19   https://www.nhs.uk/conditions/sjogrens-syndrome/

Don't

- Smoke.
- Spend too long in smoky, dry, dusty, windy places, and, if possible give air-conditioned or heated rooms a miss.
- Use deodorants and perfumed products in and around your vagina and in your bath.
- Eat too much sugary or salty food such as crisps and drink, such as fizzy drinks.
- Read, watch television or look at screens for long periods as they make you blink less and dry out your eyes so take regular breaks.

E

Eating

WHEN YOU EAT IS JUST as important as *WHAT* you eat. Most of us have been brought up on three meals a day, breakfast, lunch and dinner, and this habit dies hard. But there are several reasons why this regularity may not suit you and you find yourself eating when you're not really hungry. We should all avoid that if possible. And then there's the myth that breakfast is the most important meal of the day, and it is for the people whose work involves great physical effort. And it should be said, children up to the age of 11 or 12 should have breakfast because they're active, need calories, and there's school to navigate each morning.

But quite a number of people don't feel like eating first thing and if you're one of them you shouldn't feel dragooned into eating when you don't want to. If you're one of the people who, like me, feels no desire for food in the morning we're lucky because we have a ready-made timetable that shortens our eating window. What I mean is, if you eat your last meal of the day, say at 7-7:30pm then only eat again at say, 12-1pm the next day when you've gone 16-17 hours without eating. Some people call this fasting but it isn't really a serious fast, it's just lengthening the time between meals.

Your body loves it and there are many benefits from narrowing your eating window up until the age of about 75. After that always discuss it with your doctor as you might go short of essential nourishment. What's so good about narrowing your eating window? First of all, your metabolism can take a rest, second your hormones can align into a healthy pattern and iron out peaks of blood sugar so your insulin stays low and steady. That way you avoid craving food. A third thing is you give your brain a rest and it then has the capacity to do some housekeeping. After about 12-13 hours without food your brain can turn its attention to the important task of getting rid of rubbish. It does this by breaking down brain cells that are past their sell-by date (apoptosis) while retaining anything useful the cell may contain. So it helps brain health, even rejuvenation, by unclogging the brain.

But perhaps the greatest pay-off of narrowing your eating window is it can cure, yes cure, type 2 diabetes. It does this by preventing raised blood sugar levels, the first step on the slippery slope to type 2 diabetes. So your blood sugar levels stay in the normal range. Insulin levels swing down to the normal range too and your appetite is controlled. Most importantly, you lose weight. A few years ago research proving this concept was published and the crucial number of hours without food was 14[20]. All the people in the study who were able to refrain from eating lost a lot of weight and were cured of type 2 diabetes. Their vulnerability to heart disease, strokes and cancer disappeared too. I found the research irresistible and started to eat in the pattern the research advocated. For me, missing out on breakfast was the easiest way to build a 14-hour gap in my eating but it can be any meal that's easy for you.

So does "fasting" do you good?

My answer is an unequivocal yes. The first time I came across fasting was in research done by Professor Tim Spector, a

---

[20] https://www.kcl.ac.uk/news/14-hour-fasting-improves-hunger-mood-sleep

formidable scientist. In a nutshell he and his team showed people with type 2 diabetes benefit greatly from fasting because it makes you insulin sensitive and that brings your blood pressure down. This in itself can prevent some of the long-term complications of diabetes.

I was so convinced by the research I devised my own "fasting" plan on the basis of what's good for diabetes is good enough for me.

Intermittent fasting became fashionable in the shape of the 5:2 diet where you eat normally for five days but on the other two you only eat 500 calories. The first thing that happens is you take in fewer calories. The second important change is you're restricting your eating time. Personally, I don't think this kind of fasting is as radical as the notion we have of cutting out most of our food. Restricting eating time is cutting down on your eating window. You feed your body less often and you do this by stretching the time between meals once every 24 hours.

My personal plan for healthy eating

The plan encompasses two guiding principles: first, you needn't think, as we've all thought, breakfast is the most important meal of the day (Spector again), so if you want you can skip it. Second, you can extend the time between meals by dropping the meal of your choice.

So to get started I dropped breakfast and I stopped eating after 7pm. The first time I eat is at around 1pm for lunch the next day. That means I only take in food for six hours a day. I not only enjoy it, it does me good. I favour this way of eating because we evolved to eat this way. As hunter-gatherers we were used to eating only once in 24 hours. Surprisingly, your body enjoys not eating because it can rest and while it's resting it can pay attention to the important job of repairing itself. Gene repair is very important.

Our genes have the tendency to mutate, causing disease. But we have a built-in repair system – mutations are chopped out before they can do harm and the gene is restored to its healthy state. Without this repair system cancer genes will flourish and cause mayhem.

Paradoxically, restricted eating controls appetite because it lowers your levels of ghrelin, the hunger hormone so you want to eat not just less food but less often. (By the way, this is exactly how weight loss drugs work.) Your body is depleted of glucose and then there's the bonus that you'll lose weight because after not eating for 12+ hours your body burns fat instead.

The medical benefits of my eating plan are legion: lower insulin, lower blood pressure, improved gut function, increased effectiveness of cancer treatments and boosting several anti-ageing pathways.

Why would I not skip breakfast?

Fasting may protect against inflammation

Scientists working in Cambridge have shown fasting reduces inflammation.[21] Inflammation in the body caused by an errant immune system, is at the root of many chronic diseases such as type 2 diabetes, heart disease and cancer.

Fasting controls hunger and improves mood and sleep

If you're prepared to restrict your eating window to around 14 hours, any 14 hours, you'll have higher energy, better mood, lower hunger levels and better sleep.

Try not to vary your eating window. Consistency brings the most benefits.

---

21   https://www.cam.ac.uk/research/news/scientists-identify-how-fasting-may-protect-against-inflammation

Dr Miriam Stoppard

Exercise Is Everything

AS I SIT HERE WRITING, the headline in *the Guardian* says: "Exercise 'better than drugs' to stop cancer returning after treatment". I feel I could rest my case now. Here's why.

- Your heart and your lungs love exercise because it increases their efficiency and so you can be more active.
- Your body loves being supple and mobile and having great stamina.
- Your body loves exercise because it lowers cholesterol and so you're less likely to have heart attacks or strokes.
- Your body loves exercise because you have better balance and so fewer falls.
- Your body loves exercise because it helps you sleep better.
- Your bones love exercise so you get less osteoporosis.
- You love exercise because it increases the amount of endorphins in your blood so you have an eight-hour high after exercise.
- Your anxiety and depression are less when you exercise because exercise hormones lower the need for antidepressants.
- Your blood pressure loves exercise because it's lower.
- Your appetite loves exercise because it's regulated and stops you having cravings and binges.
- Your gut likes exercise because it helps irritable bowel syndrome (IBS).
- You love exercise because it can reshape your body.
- Your brain loves exercise because the growth hormones produced during exercise make new brain cells, so cognitive thinking and memory improve.

- You love exercise because it's good for migraine and cures headaches.

How to start exercising

When starting to exercise, take it slowly and gently. Over 60s have to be kind to their bodies because we have neither the strength nor the stamina we used to. As a safety precaution, always check with your doctor to make sure you're strong enough to start on an exercise programme.

- If your aim is to exercise in the long-term, choose something you really like otherwise you won't stick at it.
- If you don't look forward to your exercises and feel they're a chore, you're probably doing the wrong ones and should look around for something else.
- Bear in mind that if you feel the exercises are punishing, you're probably pushing yourself too hard, so throttle back.
- Your exercise should be at a level when you can carry on a conversation. If you can't, the exercise you're doing is too strenuous for you.
- The best kind of exercise is one that fits into your daily routine, like walking to the shops, taking the dog for a walk, taking the stairs rather than taking the lift.
- Exercising after a full meal is asking for trouble. Your heart probably finds it difficult to cope with digesting food and pumping a good blood supply to your muscles so give your heart a chance, wait until at least an hour and a half after you've eaten, more if it's a big meal.
- Aim to progress slowly and gradually. Don't be tempted to up the distance or the speed you walk before you're ready.
- Once you're happy with the level of fitness you've reached, slow down a little in order to maintain that level.

Remember, just increasing the amount of walking you're doing will increase your fitness. To my mind it's better to exercise gently every day than to exercise strenuously three times a week.

But if you're a weekend warrior who can only fit in exercise on a Saturday and Sunday that's good enough. Research has shown that people can be as fit exercising only at the weekend as they can working out frequently during the week[22].

Exercise in a chair? Yes you can...

There are many exercise programmes on YouTube should you wish to join in a session, some of them are quite short like 15 minutes and would involve about 10-12 exercises, each taking 30 seconds with a 10-second rest in between. I recommend that you go on to YouTube (put in the search bar something like "chair exercises for older people") and take a look at these programmes until you find one that suits you. If you can, do one each morning. My favourite one starts with exercises for the feet and then works up gradually to the top of the body. For each exercise 10-12 reps are enough.

First of all, make sure your chair is safe and stable and you can sit comfortably on it. There are three different positions for doing exercises. Position 1: sitting to the back of the chair, Position 2: sit to the centre of the chair and Position 3: towards the front of the chair. In all these positions make sure you're balanced and safe.

Sitting down, the first one is leg extensions where you swing alternate legs forwards and back from the knee.

Then there are straight leg lifts where you lift your leg up till it's straight, hold, then lower.

Next lift the heels off the floor, it's really good for your calves.

Then the opposite movement, toe raising for the ankles, together or alternate right and left.

---

22   https://www.massgeneral.org/news/press-release/weekend-warrior-physical-activity-heart-benefits

Then there are side taps where you rotate one leg to the side and then the other leg to the side.

Moving up the body to the abdomen do twists, keeping the shoulders down and your head in line with your spine. Twist your body from the waist around to the right and move your head as far as you can then bring your body back to the centre, twist to the left, turn as far as you can and then back to centre.

The next exercise is very simple. Sitting with good posture, you stretch your arms alternately down to either side to reach your heels.

Next, raise your arms together to shoulder level from by your side then alternate arm reaches, taking your hand from the side of your body and reaching up as far as you can with alternate arms.

Next is the biceps curl where you flex your elbow and reach with your hand up to your shoulder, which you can do simply with your arm, or you can hold, for instance, a can of beans in each hand to increase the workload and the effort you have to make.

Then from your arms down by your sides lift them above your shoulders straight and reach as high as you can.

Then arm pulls with your arms raised and your hands touching, pull them back so that you feel the shoulder stretch and the shoulder blades come together.

If you feel inclined, you could go on to exercises for your heart, the first of which is to march with your feet, arms by your side. The second is to march and swing your arms as well, and the third is to stand up from your chair without holding on to anything, simply using your quads, say 15 times.

Here's a YouTube channel that I find quite helpful, and you might too: Elder Fit TV (www.youtube.com/@elderfitTV).

My final thoughts on exercising safely

Exercises should never be a chore. If they are, you're doing the wrong ones.

The best kind of exercise is one that fits in with your daily life, like cycling to work or going to the shops, or taking the dog for a walk, climbing stairs rather than taking the lift and doing a bit of exercise wherever you are, even while working at the kitchen sink.

Please don't think that you need to spend a lot of money on expensive equipment. You can do all the exercises you need without buying anything.

Always check how fit you are before you start on any exercise programme. If you're in doubt about your fitness, check with your doctor.

Don't be overzealous about increasing the length of your exercises too quickly. Slowly and surely is the way to go. You could always check your pulse rate so that you reach the level of fitness suitable for your age over a period of weeks, and that should never be less than six weeks.

It's worth emphasising again, you need to choose activities and exercises that you enjoy. If you don't, you'll never stick to your exercise programme. You should never find exercises physically punishing. If they are, you're probably pushing yourself too hard.

I know I'm repeating myself but it really is unwise to exercise on a full stomach, best to wait for an hour or so before starting on strenuous exercise and try doing a warm-up before you begin.

To maintain your level of fitness try working out three times a week.

F

Falls

I'M SURE YOU KNOW OF an old person having a fall and being admitted as an emergency to hospital. After a fall some people may have to move from their own home to a care home for their safety.

About a third of people (2.5 million) aged 65 and above, and about half of people aged 80 will fall at least once a year. Falls can be very serious, causing a fracture that needs hospitalisation. Falls and fractures in the over 65s take up over four million hospital bed days per year in England alone, at an estimated cost of £2 billion[23].

In older age deteriorating vision, dizziness, unsteady gait, less mobile joints and stiff muscles all contribute to falls.

My key advice is: be alert. It seems falls involving old people occur at a particular time of day – between 6am and noon which corresponds to the morning ritual of getting up and out of bed and dressing. Falls tail off in the afternoon hours when many people are resting. There's a moderate increase between 5pm and 9pm, dinner time and going to bed. A third of falls occur during the night when trying to get out of bed but 1 in 6 are just reaching for something on the bedside table. More than half are while walking to the bathroom.

---

23   https://ukhsa.blog.gov.uk/2014/07/17/the-human-cost-of-falls/

Preventing falls

Falls are the number one cause of injuries in the home. Children under five and adults over 70 are the most vulnerable. Important factors are:

- **Rugs** are a big tripping hazard for young and old people. Ask yourself: do you really need that rug? If not, get rid of it. At the very least, tape or tack them to the floor.
- **Stairs.** Remove clutter from stairs and walkways. Stairs should have handrails, preferably on both sides and good lighting.
- Keep all **cables** out of places where you walk.
- **Lights.** Good lighting is essential. Have night-lights in bedrooms, bathrooms, and halls.
- **Bathroom.** Install grab-bars and non-slip mats in the bath or shower. Clean up any water that splashes on floors straight away.

My routine for getting up after a fall

About a year ago I fell five times in one week, badly bruising my arm and leg and I decided to take myself in hand and pay more attention to where I was walking.

So, I started to look for "edges" which is one of the first things we stop seeing with clarity as we get older, the edge of a pavement, the edge of a step, the edge of stairs, an uneven paving stone. I also stopped turning quickly and started moving around slowly one step at a time so that I didn't swing around. I haven't fallen since.

Any fall takes it out of you so stay still and collect yourself. Take note of anywhere that's hurting or is painful when you move it. Keep still. Just rest and take slow, deep breaths so that you can do a complete check of your body and wait till you feel able to move. This may take four or five minutes.

The first thing I do is to turn prone, onto my front. Then I raise my upper body on my arms with my hands about the same distance apart as my shoulders. I check everything to make sure that I feel okay and ready to go onto the next step.

The next thing I do is to draw my legs one at a time underneath me so that I'm kneeling. When I'm kneeling safely on all fours I rest for a minute or two before I contemplate the next move.

I then pull one of my legs (the stronger of my two legs) underneath my body so that I'm still resting on two hands, one knee and one foot.

I then press up hard on my toe that's on the ground, at the same time taking the weight of my upper body on my bent knee by pressing down.

If I'm lucky enough and strong enough, this gets me to my feet.

By the way, I don't hesitate to ask for help if there's anyone near me when I attempt this manoeuvre, and nor should you. Never be embarrassed by the onward march of your body's frailty.

As I've got older I have a tendency to shuffle. I developed an increasing tendency to fall, usually by tripping over an uneven pavement and this is because, as with many other people my age, I don't lift my feet clear of the ground. I decided, after that series of five falls in quick succession, that I'd have to retrain myself to walk by lifting my feet further off the ground. I manage this about half the time. In the other half I still trip but not as severely as before and I stay upright.

I also protect myself against lying helpless after falling by wearing a smart watch which is programmed to ask me, when it detects a fall, if I need help and it phones my emergency contact. I would recommend having a smart watch to anyone who stumbles. If you choose you can have an alarm button on a watch or around your neck connected to a subscription service should you fall and need help.

Dr Miriam Stoppard

Family

NO MATTER WHAT HAPPENS TO our society, I hope fervently the family survives. Change it will, but to my mind it's the group that keeps us cemented together. Not least because it nurtures human beings at both ends of life. It has persisted intact through Biblical times and the Egyptian, Greek, and Roman civilisations and through the medieval ages.

The industrial revolution, however, led to new configurations as families left the land to settle and work in cities, urbanisation. Since then, the greatest changes have been between the roles of mothers and fathers which started to overlap after the industrial revolution and became equal with the parent-child relationship remaining paramount. The nuclear family (mother, father and children) is the oldest kind of family in existence. It may swell to accommodate other siblings and grandparents and sometimes includes children who have married, their spouse's children from an earlier relationship (the extended family).

In this form the family provides love, security and companionship to all its members. Within it, children are reared and needy members are looked after. It provides the most basic needs of food, clothing, shelter and physical security. It may also steer standards of sexual conduct.

Family rules tend to promote order and stability in society as a whole. In the modern family, members no longer live in the family unit for as long as adults, generally moving out in their late teens as they set off for work or university. The present day cost of housing does, however, mean more adult children live at home for longer than previous decades.

But there are always pressures on families. Involvement in wars often breaks up families. Divorce is another factor. Divorce has existed for millennia, and across faiths there has been recognition that some marriages don't survive.

The wonderful song 'We are Family' reflects another form of family altogether – groups of people united by a common philosophy and culture such as that which encompasses the LGBTQ+ community. Family is also a mechanism for inheritance, be it land, assets or money. In the UK we still have the aristocratic but outdated primogeniture where the total inheritance goes to the eldest son and the rest of the family has to fend for itself.

I think we can be optimistic about the future of family because I really believe families will support elderly relatives and where that kind of care is given, it's a far greater contribution to the well-being of older family members than can be provided by the NHS. I never cease to be impressed by how the younger generation takes care of the older generation, especially daughters, though my sons think about my needs and make sure they're met by taking better care of me than I ever expected. One of my sons, Will, started to put his hand under my elbow to guide me across busy roads when I was in my early 60s and I realised there had been a role reversal – he was taking care of me, rather than my taking care of him. So I asked him, "Will, can you remember when you first felt you needed to take care of me, rather than my taking care of you?" He didn't miss a beat, "Oh, when I was about five years old, Mum."

Within families various members can visit, go for a walk, treat an older person to a meal out, arrange a cinema visit and enjoy a sports event together. Something which I never thought would happen to me and might similarly surprise other grandparents like me, is that my grandchildren are always in touch with me and visit me often. My favourite word in the English language is granny.

Older people, at a time when they really need stability and

continuity, can be confronted by family upheaval on account of divorce, remarriage, new relations with various children and children-in-law. They can be challenged having to face up to changing relationships with sons and daughters-in-law of whom they're very fond, with the added strain of having to decide with whom and near whom they're going to live. This reconstitution of the family with changing relationships can prove difficult for older members. Looking at it a different way, grandparents may have a crucial role to play in divorce. To a child whose mum and dad are going their separate ways, a grandparent can be a rock they can rely on. There's even special legislation for grandparents to apply to the courts for custody of grandchildren when one or both parents have died.

Grandparents' rights after the death of a parent[24]

Grandparents don't have automatic rights to gain custody of a grandchild whose parent has died, nor do they have an automatic right to apply for custody of their grandchild; they must get permission first. Before applying to the court, grandparents normally have to attend a Mediation Information and Assessment Meeting (MIAM) to explore whether the matter can be resolved outside court through mediation.

The next step is to seek permission from the Family Court to make an application by completing a C100 form along with a request for permission. This application can be completed and submitted online.

In some cases, grandparents may apply for a Special Guardianship Order (SGO). An SGO gives the grandparents parental responsibility and allows them to make significant decisions about the child's upbringing while maintaining the child's legal relationship with their birth parents.

---

24   https://reissedwards.co.uk/family-law-blog/who-gets-custody-of-the-child-if-a-parent-dies/

Can grandparents get custody of their grandchildren?[25]

They can in certain situations where parents are unable to care for their children. Grandparents obtain temporary or permanent custody, which is also known as special or legal guardianship. Grandparents also have the option of adopting their grandchildren in special circumstances.

The courts will always consider the wellbeing of a child when coming to a decision which focuses on a child and in some scenarios grandparents may be best placed to care for their grandchildren.

With grandparents becoming younger all the time and children increasingly having close relationships with their grandparents, the option of grandparent custody doesn't seem such a bad idea.

Fitness – How Fit Are You?

I'VE SAID IT BEFORE, BEING fit is different from being healthy. For instance, you can run 5K, do 30 press-ups and cycle for an hour, but you could also have a high cholesterol or be pre-diabetic. Most of this book is to do with being healthy as we get older but I just want to say something here about what our expectations for fitness might be as we go through our 60s, 70s and 80s, and what we should be aiming for.

---

25 https://www.kabirfamilylaw.co.uk/grandparents-rights/#:~:text=As%20mentioned%20grandparents%20do%20not,not%20letting%20grandparents%20see%20grandchildren

60s

The most important thing to remember is it's never too late to start paying attention to fitness so it doesn't matter whether you've been working at your fitness all through your life or you haven't. Some people would say in order to decide how fit you are, you should do the "old man" test. Never done it myself, but it's said to be a good indicator of your functional strength, balance, coordination, and flexibility. I think the reason I haven't attempted it so far is that I know I should fail because I'm unable to balance standing on one leg for any length of time, especially if I'm trying to do something with the other leg. The old man test involves you standing on one leg while you put on a sock and a shoe on the other leg. You also tie the laces of the shoe. If you can do that with both legs then in my book you are pretty fit!

If the old man test is beyond you, you could try something gentler by standing on one foot and then the other when you're brushing your teeth or when you're at the sink, or when you stand to take a phone call. Tai Chi is good for balance. You might also like to try some isometric exercises, such as doing a wall sit for 45 seconds while your legs are at 90° in a "chair squat" leaning against the wall. Doing small things as you go through the day will also make a contribution to your functional fitness. It's said these eccentric movements done through the day can be transformative as we get older. Eccentric movements are exercises which aim to lengthen a muscle, for instance, doing push-ups and bicep curls. So if you practise throughout the day lowering yourself into a squat, you have the benefits of lengthening your muscles which it's claimed can transform your ageing life. There's good evidence for this, in the shape of a recent study that found just five minutes of eccentric exercise can improve strength, flexibility and mental health in sedentary adults in just four weeks[26]. Keep up the gardening if you're a gardener, and short, sharp bursts of anything manual involving using your muscles and working them hard. This practice is good for our strength at every age.

70s

If you haven't got any resistance bands, now's the time to get them. You can buy them in any local sports shop or online. They're the key to strength training which is one of the most effective age-related interventions there is. Strength training can be with weights, resistance bands or simply body weight. It's important because it's been shown to significantly decrease your risk of falling. It also increases walking speed, tissue regeneration and lowers the frequency of fractures and disability. But as with other aspects of physical fitness, it also improves our mental fitness by boosting something called "brain-derived neurotrophic factor" which importantly improves memory and combats cognitive decline. So, what do you do with your resistance bands? What I do is to hold one end under my foot and do chest pulls, biceps curls, leg press, and bent over rows. I try to do three sessions a week. I can't do any more because I need to recover between sessions. If you're using weights, start with ones you can comfortably lift 10-15 times, but first go online and see how it's done properly by a trainer. Once you feel comfortable with those weights you can increase them by a kilo (c. 2lbs) or so. You can buy a cheap starter set on Amazon[27].

Want to know how fit you are right now? Well, try sitting on a kitchen chair and with your hands crossed across your chest stand up and sit down as often as you can for 30 seconds. If you reach 14/15, you're fit enough.

---

26   https://pubmed.ncbi.nlm.nih.gov/40131475/
27   https://www.amazon.co.uk/

80s

When I saw the criteria for being fit in your 80s, I laughed out loud. The first one is to walk unaided for 10 minutes. My usual walks are longer than a mile and I haven't yet resorted to the use of a stick unless I'm feeling very wobbly, which fortunately hasn't happened for 12 months. But if you can walk unaided for 10 minutes, you're in good nick. The balance test for us in our 80s is less taxing than the one in our 70s. All you have to do is to lift a foot an inch or two off the floor and keep it there for 10 seconds then repeat with the other foot. If you can do this you're pretty fit for your age. And you can do more resistance band exercises, only gentler ones than those in your 70s. Do some seated rows, side steps and overhead side bends. If you can add a short walk to this every day, that's great. In the 80s two thirds of all injury-related deaths are due to falls, therefore it's important if we can prevent them. Something like yoga or pilates with low impact, twice weekly if you can, will reward you with continued independence and confidence in what your body can do for you.

Fractures

FRACTURES IN OLDER PEOPLE ARE different from those sustained by younger people. For one thing the bone tends to break nearer a joint and in a younger person it's the bone shaft that breaks. After the menopause when oestrogen levels drop in women, they're more likely to experience fractures than men, especially near the wrist, of the hip, and the vertebrae in the spine.

A fracture of the hip depends on how strong the thigh bone is, the top of which forms the hip joint. Often it's brittle because of osteoporosis. One in five women, and 40% of women with a fractured hip, have osteopenia, the stage before osteoporosis where the bone softens due to too little calcium in them. It may happen as early as your 40s.

Here's something interesting: Osteopenia is greatest in the months of February to April, and lowest in the months October to December. The theory is this difference is due to the seasonal variation in the hours of sunshine when the skin can make vitamin D. Vitamin D helps the body absorb calcium from food and deposit it in our bones. As we get older, it's vitamin D and calcium we need to keep our bones healthy. Both osteopenia and osteoarthritis show up on bone density scans.

Fractured wrists are uncommon in adults but there's a steep rise after the menopause in women. This is due to loss of oestrogen from menopause onwards, and it can be corrected with HRT. Crush fractures of the vertebrae become more and more common as we age due to osteoporosis and may cause compression of the spinal bones. A curved spine (Dowager's Hump) and loss of height may result. A lot of people aren't aware of it but something as simple as regular weight-bearing exercise like walking every day will protect you against osteopenia as well as osteoporosis. It's useful to know that walking stimulates your body to absorb all the calcium you eat as well as all the vitamin D in an attempt to keep the bones sturdy and strong.

Future Fears

MOST OF US HAVE FELT what can be described as existential anxiety at various points during our lives. It's a normal part of being human, realising that life is ultimately uncertain. This kind of anxiety can arise during times of flux in our lives, during transitions from one phase of our lives to another and when change is thrust upon us and the future seems unknown. This existential anxiety brings with it a feeling of unease, dread, apprehension with thoughts of death, even of suicide. Existential dread is a deepening of these anxieties with worries about failure, about life's meaning, life's purpose and mortality. It's nearly always accompanied by despair about the human condition when we're plagued by questions about the meaning of life, free will, identity, purpose and mortality and people are asking them earlier and earlier.

I don't know about you but I can't remember the labels given to various generations of people and the timelines they fit into so, in case you do too, I've drawn up a list of them with dates.

- **The Greatest Generation:** 1901-1927
- **The Silent Generation:** 1928-1945
- **Baby Boomers:** 1946-1964
- **Generation X:** 1965-1980
- **Millennials/Generation Y:** 1981-1996
- **Generation Z:** 1997-2012
- **Generation Alpha:** 2013-2025
- **Generation Beta**: 2025-2039

It would seem these existential questions preoccupy younger generations who are asking them at a much earlier age than previous generations. That's to their credit and we oldies should sympathise with them. We only need to look around the world and see so much conflict, hatred, wilful cruelty, the danger of nuclear war, the destruction of the earth's ecology, exploitation, racial and religious hate. If you're a woman there's more angst, what it means to be female, what it means to be queer, what it means to be a single mother, what it means to be the subject of sexism or abuse.

The irrationality of our leaders and the demagoguery practised by extremist right governments makes women feel powerless and despairing.

There's always a glimmer of hope though, and we can find reasons to be optimistic. For instance, I have infinite faith in medical researchers to come up with new ways of treating diseases, new ways of preventing diseases and new ways of diagnosing them. Alongside hope, there's love. At the end of our lives, we realise there's nothing more important in life than love. And if we're wise, we shall take the opportunity to grasp it, embrace it, and feel its joy. I've concluded that joy itself is an antidote to these anxieties, dreads and despair that may overwhelm us now and then. So I look for joy and if I find it, I bathe in it. It's calming, it's nourishing, it's inspiring, and I would say it's as great a life force as exercise or eating well or any of the other ways we are encouraged to practise in order to stay healthy. In respect of this I would say older people who are comfortable with their feelings could set an example to the younger generation by being open about their emotions and expressing them fully.

If at any time you find yourself in the throes of feeling overcome by the uncertainty of life there are some well-accepted coping strategies.

Accept that anxiety and worry are a natural part of the human experience and not all questions have answers, even putting trust in yourself to make things better.

Meaning, which we can find in our values and things which are important to us, giving a sense of purpose and feeling less lonely.

Create something, and it needn't be a huge undertaking. It can be something as simple as appreciating creativity in others, helping you to explore your emotions and find meaning in what you feel.

Meditation, breathing and mindfulness, can bring your mind back to the present, making it possible to absorb yourself in what's going on around you at that precise moment, and therefore avoiding uncertainties.

To believe that we're **not defined** by existential anxiety and dread. Most people feel them and we're not alone.

Practise gratitude, this is something that means a lot to me. We have so much in our lives to be grateful for, no matter how down in the dumps we're feeling. Just start counting your blessings and if you do there will be many and much to be grateful for.

Share feelings, there's absolutely no reason to hold your feelings in, letting them out and sharing them with others is a huge relief and one you should learn to practise. I'm reminded of one of my mum's favourite sayings, "A trouble shared is a trouble halved".

There's no better way **to get grounded** than to be with your grandchildren so keep relationships alive and sweet. Be a grandparent who's nice to know.

Meaningful activities will always bring you joy, and they can be volunteering, arranging a coffee morning, getting the family together, doing charity runs, in fact contributing to charities in any form.

As we get older, I think we get more reflective and it can be a balm for the soul to explore your spiritual needs and delve into different philosophies.

G

Gardening

ABOUT 24 YEARS AGO I was wandering about my garden admiring the roses which were in full bloom. Roses everywhere. The air was full of the scent of them. I was concentrating on a particular rose which I loved and I felt my mind go into free fall. I was entirely absorbed by the rose, its beauty, its habitat, and its smell. My mind was emptied of everything except the roses and what they brought to me. I stood stock still for several minutes letting that feeling flow through my brain. That's what gardening does. It feeds your mind. If you like, you can call that mindfulness. I'm a passionate gardener so I practise a lot of mindfulness.

My passion for gardening arose when my first baby was due. As part of my nesting instinct, I wanted to make his birthplace as beautiful as possible. The house in which I was living with my husband and two stepsons had a large garden but completely untended. I was in the third trimester by the time I had the thought that I wanted to prepare my baby's home for his arrival. In the spring the only plants I could find to adorn his birthplace were annuals and potted plants. I filled the borders with pink and white geraniums, petunias and spring flowers. As it was a large garden I had to work very hard indeed, spending quite a lot of time bending down to which my mother would shout, "Miriam, stand up. If you go on bending like that you'll harm your baby's spine."

It isn't true of course, it's just an old wives' tale.

Speak to any gardener and they, like me, will find it difficult to put into words what makes them so enamoured of gardening. Yes, of course it's got to do with encouraging new life, tending to young plants and making sure they have everything they need, designing your plantings, and making sure that there is something in flower for the whole year including the cold winter months, and feeding your family with fruit and veg. But most of all I think it's to do with the way flowers, shrubs and plants reward you. They ask for so little, yet every year come back with glorious displays of flowers that make you weep.

I particularly love how plants intermingle with each other in ways you could never have anticipated or planned for. And all the while, of course, gardening is good for you. I've already mentioned how it can be therapeutic and ease your anxieties and pain. The punctuation of the seasons each year is very reassuring and calming. But also pottering around the garden is good for your physical health. The longest living people on the planet, the Okinawans, potter all day, they're always on their feet and keep moving. Well, a spell in the garden will do the same for you while nourishing your brain and your emotions.

If you don't have a garden you can express your nurturing instincts by having a window box and inspect it daily, even talk to your plants. I talk to mine all the time.

Giddiness

AS WE GET OLDER, GIDDINESS or vertigo is one of the most common symptoms we have to cope with. Women are more likely to be affected than men and quite often a cause isn't found. Some factors like wax in the ears, ear disease, high and low blood pressure, also some drugs like painkillers and antibiotics are linked to giddiness.

Vertigo, deafness and Meniere's disease, which is more common in men over the age of about 45 or 50 are also linked. Meniere's disease is a violent type of giddiness in deaf people with the feeling of spinning and being sick. Even the smallest movement is unbearable. It's due to disease in the balancing organ of the inner ear and can be treated with new drugs from your doctor.

Girlfriends – I Don't Know What I'd Do Without Them

I BELONG TO A WHATSAPP GROUP of about eight women of a similar age, similar disposition and similar way of life. We share a lot of common ground, having grandchildren, some of us are widows or live alone, some of us have chronic ill health and few of us enjoy total good health. We're concerned about Covid boosters, about schools and unis for grandchildren, and staying fit as we get older. Some of us have a long shared history. Two of the founder members I've known for almost 40 years, so we have a lot of shared baggage, shared joys and shared concerns. I wish every woman had a group of such girlfriends, always there when I need support, a shoulder to lean on, and a problem to solve. And despite our many similarities, it's the differences in our backgrounds and life experiences which means their advice often comes from a different viewpoint to my own. We're so comfortable with each other, last year we even went on a trip to Ibiza together, including one friend in a wheelchair due to multiple sclerosis, as the guests of our oldest member who is now only a year from being 100. Together we can attempt anything and overcome every obstacle. We do feel strong. We give each other strength.

I had an interesting experience when we arrived at Ibiza airport. I was standing at the carousel waiting for my luggage when I felt some arms go around my waist and a beery voice said, "See you at the rave then". I turned round and found the red face of one of the passengers on our plane who'd started his trip to Ibiza by celebrating on the journey out. It was my rear view with long hair, dressed in holiday clothes that gave him the false impression I was fair game. On seeing my 80+ face, however, his arms dropped immediately and he backed off. The hazards of travelling – even with a group of friends.

I'm very comfortable with the friends I have and rarely feel inclined to make new ones. These days there's always the option of making friends via the internet and many people do, successfully, though the less techie among us might find it daunting. Making new friends requires a leap of faith to overcome fear of rejection. At our age, we shouldn't let that stop us. You can start up a conversation anywhere. If someone joins you on a park bench you can strike up a conversation with something like, "I love this park, don't you?", or "The daffodils here were amazing this year. Did you see them?" or, "Aren't the trees wonderful here?". Sitting next to another granny at the school play it's easy to start chatting – about grandchildren and education and what a great school it is. Given your common ground, you may find you'd like to make more of the conversation and see each other again. So I'm a great believer in "getting talking". We have social genes and we don't lose them as we get older. If anything, with the loss of inhibitions and a degree of self-confidence, we can get talking in many unlikely situations, even to a shop assistant and a taxi driver. Chat oils the wheels of life.

Of course, you'll probably make friends all the sooner if you belong to or join a group of people who are interested in the same thing – walkers, potters, singers, bridge players, chess players (I've got interested in chess since watching a series of programmes on TV and I've decided I'm going to take lessons to learn to play chess. Several of my grandchildren are good at it and I think they would enjoy a challenge from their granny, and undoubtedly would win. It seems to me a good way to share a new bond with my grandchildren as we both get older).

An important element of all the best friendships is laughter but closeness is high on the list and sharing some of life's big events is a surefire way to get closer to a friend or a relative. Your attending graduation and prize giving is something your grandchildren will never forget. Sharing any of life's milestones is richly rewarding. Even if you only do it every five or 10 years, a big get-together with friends and family will strengthen your existing relationships, and it's fertile ground for making strong new attachments. One of the payoffs is you'll boost your sense of who you are, essential if you're going to make the most of your precious advancing years.

Why friends are important for long life

Why are friends so important as you get older? Look no further than the Okinawans, the longest living race on the planet and after learning about their lifestyle I started trying to live my life their way. The changes I made are very simple to accommodate in everyday life and one had particular meaning for me. The Okinawans lean on strong family and community support. In other words, they treasure friends. Not virtual "friends" on Facebook or Twitter but real face to face friends that you can count on. This prompted me to really look after my relationships with family and girlfriends to nourish, support and comfort me.

According to a book, *The Village Effect* by Susan Pinker, the Okinawans have been doing it right for millennia. She emphasises the life-enhancing effect of friends is especially important to women. We know that people who live alone have shorter lives and that's because the human brain evolved at a time when living in cooperating groups was essential for survival. And that's one of the reasons why we women, who put a premium on deep social connections, live longer than men.

Those social connections add years to your life. Research shows that playing cards once a week or meeting friends for coffee can add as many years to your life as giving up a 20-cigarette-a-day habit. MRI scans have proved the body recovers faster after illness because an active social life boosts the immune system[28].

The alternative is bleak. Loneliness kills as this dramatic research reveals. In a study of 3,000 Californian women with breast cancer, scientists found those with a large network of friends were four times more likely to recover than those who were lonely[29]. Reaching out to other women releases oxytocin, the "love" hormone that soothes pain and lifts our spirits. It reinforces the commitment we feel to the people close to us.

People living alone are deprived of attention, affection, hugs and eye contact that we've evolved because we need them. It's biological. We've also developed what psychologists call 'reciprocal altruism', people are kind and supportive without being asked because they know they'll get it in return. The Okinawans again. This culture of being committed to family and friends is our natural and deeply programmed way of life and we go without it at our peril.

What's more, it's reinforced by body chemistry because when we

---

28   https://www.health.harvard.edu/mind-and-mood/even-a-little-socializing-is-linked-to-longevity
https://pubmed.ncbi.nlm.nih.gov/18222382/
29   https://divisionofresearch.kaiserpermanente.org/kaiser-permanente-study-shows-women-with-more-social-connections-have-higher-breast-cancer-survival-rates/

perform acts of kindness for other people, feelgood hormones like endorphins cascade through our bodies. And we live longer.

How to nurture meaningful friendships

We often choose our friends by gravitating towards people with similar views, interests and temperament. Losing touch with friends and meeting new people is part of the ebb and flow of life but there are things you can do to keep a treasured friendship going.

Put the effort in
> This doesn't mean you have to be together all the time but meeting up regularly and sharing important life events will strengthen friendships.

Plan activities you both enjoy
> Sharing a hobby or a passion for something will add an extra layer to your friendship and strengthen your bond.

Resolve conflicts
> Don't leave an argument unresolved or, as my mother used to say, "Never let the sun set on your wrath". If you disagree, try to sit down and discuss it, don't let it fester. Making up after an argument will show you both how important the other person is.

Encourage each other
> Having a supportive friend who keeps you accountable will make achieving your goals easier and vice versa. So while focusing on self-development, whether it's getting into shape, learning a new skill or moving up the ladder at work, stay in touch.

And one more thing. Not all friendships are meant to last. Sometimes you just have to let it go.

Glaucoma

GLAUCOMA IS AN URGENT MATTER at any age because if left untreated it may cause blindness. It's most prevalent in people in their 70s and 80s and is due to increased pressure inside the eye itself, usually because of fluid building up. Fluid in the eye is constantly circulating, so it drains from the eye all the time. If this drainage is blocked, more and more fluid accumulates and raises the pressure within the eyeball. Without a diagnosis and treatment it may damage the optic nerve, which carries images from the back of the eye to the back of the brain, causing blindness. Glaucoma becomes more common with age and people of African, Caribbean or Asian origin are at high risk.

If glaucoma comes on slowly there are rarely any symptoms but occasionally onset is sudden and the symptoms can be quite dramatic. There may be pain within the eye sufficient to cause nausea and vomiting, the eye is red and you may have a headache. It's a classic case of "red eye". Glaucoma is easier to diagnose when it produces rings around lights and your vision becomes blurred. So if you have any suspicious symptoms, see your GP or an optician for a check. On the other hand if you suddenly develop a painful red eye go to A&E as soon as possible. If there's an eye hospital in your area, go there. They'll have an eye A&E and you'll get prompt treatment from an eye specialist.

If you make a routine appointment to see an optician, you can have an eye test which will reveal early glaucoma in which case you should have an eye test every two years. This way treatment can be started early and prevent damage to the optic nerve. If you're found to have glaucoma, there are several treatments available to you. The first is eye drops, which will relieve your pain and help to reduce the pressure in your eye. And then possibly laser treatment which is used to unblock drainage tubes, or lower the amount of fluid your eye produces. A third option is to have surgery which is aimed at improving the drainage of fluid out of your eye.

Gout

IF YOU HAVE GOUT YOU will certainly know about it. You may have seen cartoons of men lying in bed with one foot raised and the throbbing, red swelling of their big toe. This is the classical picture of gout which does occur more as you get older and more commonly in men. There's often a family history of gout which suggests there might be an inherited abnormality of purine metabolism, the cause of gout.

Gout is a type of arthritis with profound inflammation inside the joint. Attacks come on suddenly with intense pain, swelling, and redness, typically of the big toe but it's found in other joints. It occurs when needle-like uric acid crystals accumulate in your joint where they cause inflammation and intense pain.

Why should this happen? Uric acid crystals form in a joint when you have high levels of uric acid in your blood. Your body produces uric acid quite normally as it breaks down purines which are waste products from the metabolism of proteins. Purines do have an upside, they're essential for the formation of DNA and RNA. Purines are also found in certain foods.

Normally, when the body breaks down purines to form uric acid, it's dissolved in the blood and filtered out by the kidneys.

If excess uric acid accumulates in the blood it crystallises in the joints (gout) and may form kidney stones when the kidneys have to filter high levels of uric acid out of the blood. Uric acid accumulates in the blood either because of high purine intake or because of disturbed purine metabolism.

Foods to avoid in gout (high in purines)

Some people are more sensitive to purines than others but the following foods should be avoided if possible:

- Meats, especially organ meat like liver, kidney, game and turkey.
- Seafood like sardines, herring, mackerel, anchovies and scallops.
- Certain vegetables like spinach, green peas, lentils and chickpeas.
- Other foods would include yeast products and definitely alcohol, particularly beer because of its yeast content.

Foods low in purines, eat now and then

- Low fat dairy, milk, yoghurt and cheese.
- Fruit and veg other than those mentioned above.
- Nuts and eggs.
- Wholegrains, bread, cereal and pasta.
- Coffee, may protect against the effect of uric acid levels.

Triggers

Some people have attacks if they eat the following trigger foods:

- Beer, fortified wine like Sherry and port.
- Sugary foods, drinks and sweets.
- Processed foods.
- Organ meats, liver, kidney, sweetbreads and tripe.
- Seafoods like mussels, scallops, squid, shrimp, oysters, crab and lobster.

Treatment
First line treatment for gout is often NSAIDs (non-steroidal anti-inflammatory drugs) like ibuprofen or naproxen given throughout the day every eight hours. If the pain and swelling don't improve, steroids may be tried. For someone who's having frequent attacks and is found to have higher than normal uric acid levels in the blood, a uric acid lowering agent like allopurinol taken every day, and I mean every day, can sometimes abort attacks of gout. Another such agent would be Colchicine which your doctor will prescribe or a modern alternative, Febuxostat. As the burden of getting rid of waste uric acid falls on the kidney you should have regular renal function tests to make sure that your kidneys are up to handling the load.

GPs

DO YOU REMEMBER TV'S DR Finlay's Casebook where the friendly local doctor visited his patients in their homes and charged them a few shillings? Seems like another world. For starters home visits are often done by expert paramedics rather than overworked doctors. In truth, the whole of general practice has changed. Doctors have much larger caseloads and spend more time on admin than in the past. As a result the practice will have auxiliary staff like receptionist, nurse, pharmacist, phlebotomist and a paramedic, and possibly a physiotherapist, all of whom you may need and see in place of your GP.

Most practices have a gatekeeper, the practice manager, so your doctor may seem distant. This is heightened by many GPs opting for "tele-medical care" where you'll be seen remotely and you chat together on screen. This may not be to everyone's taste but if there's no alternative, ask a friend to be with you to help you feel confident the first time you try it. If you have difficulty getting out and about you might find online appointments far more convenient and comfortable. Whether your consultation is online or face to face it's wise to prepare for your consultation by making notes about your complaint. For example, if you're in pain be prepared to describe the type of pain, where it is, if it's constant or comes and goes, what relieves it and what makes it worse, what tests are suggested, do you require medication and what sort, possible side effects, next steps. Don't end the conversation without knowing a possible/probable diagnosis.

For a consultation with your doctor you'll feel confident if you've taken some time to prepare the main questions you want your doctor to answer for you.

I've assembled a few lists that could act as guidelines in several scenarios.

Questions to ask your doctor about medications

Choose the questions that will help you most. Have the list with you when you see the doctor, then you won't forget anything important.

- How will this medicine help me?
- Will it take a long time to act?
- Do I take it with food or on an empty stomach?
- For how many days shall I take this medicine?
- What times of day should I take it?
- My other medicines, will it affect them?
- What side effects can I expect?
- Should I contact you if I have side effects?
- Are there any foods, drinks or other medicines I shouldn't take?
- What should I do if I miss a dose?

At some point your doctor may want you to have a scan. Here are some questions to give you a bit of background.

Questions to ask your doctor if they recommend a scan

- Does this test use radiation? If so, is it safe?
- Are there any other tests that you could use? Are they risky? Is one better than the rest?
- What's this test for?
- What will it tell you?
- Would I need anaesthesia for this test? Local? General? Other?
- How will you use the results to decide on my treatment?

How to remember what the doctor told you

A consultation with a doctor can be intimidating and if you're anxious it's difficult to remember what the doctor says to you. I would always take a friend or family member who can remember and help make a list for you of the salient points.

Summon up your courage and ask questions
If you're not sure you fully understand what your doctor is saying, tell them, and your friend. Ask them to repeat it or explain everything in simpler terms.

Make sure you prepare for meeting with your doctor
Before you go make a list of all your questions and concerns, leaving space for the answers. You and your friend can make notes during the consultation.

Don't hesitate to have moral support
With a friend you'll feel more confident and they can help make sure you understand what's being discussed and what you need to do to manage your condition.

There may be times when you need to see your doctor but with practices busy and the earliest appointment you can get is several days or even weeks ahead, you don't want to bother your doctor and hesitate to make a fuss. What should you do? I think you have to enlist the support of your family. A son or daughter or even a son-in-law or daughter-in-law should take up your case with the practice and ask for an early appointment. Your relative may be able to get you an earlier appointment if they phone the practice as soon as it opens and say you need an urgent appointment.

What if I'm too ill to visit my GP?

There'll be times when you're not well enough to make it to your GP surgery. Ask your GP practice for information on how to request a home visit, then ask for one. If possible, try to call your GP in the morning if you think you need a visit the same day. Remember, if you need to see your GP but can't make it to the surgery, they must offer a home visit instead. They will factor in how urgent your condition is (triage) when arranging a home visit. Your GP might also be able to give you advice through a telephone or video consultation as an alternative. A highly trained paramedic may visit you rather than your doctor.

Grandparents/ Grandparenting

A GREAT JOY LIES IN WAIT for many of us as we get older. Grandparenthood. Becoming a grandparent is one of the most enriching phases of your life and something to look forward to and relish. I'd like to think of grandparents, and grandmothers in particular, as being the cement that keeps families together and helps provide a child with a close family group where they feel loved, valued and secure. Sometimes a grandparent can be a refuge for a troubled child.

Fortunately in our society there are lots of us, in the UK about 14 million grandparents. Stats reveal grandparents provide about two-fifths (40%) of childcare in this country. Government figures show that childcare provided by grandparents saves the economy up to a whopping £4 billion a year[30]. So I think we're justified in thinking we're valuable, not only to families but also to the smooth running of the country and the economy.

When I became a granny I discovered I could be an enabler to my grandchildren and help them to enjoy not only their interests but help them achieve their goals and ambitions. I could be a reliable source of encouragement, a kind of coach, only too pleased to take on the role of cheerleader. Someone who couldn't wait to get down on the floor to play or join in a game. To my grandchildren, however, my most important role was to give them my undivided attention so they were my sole focus, something they didn't always get from their parents who were busy with other things, whereas I wanted nothing more than to concentrate on my grandchild.

Becoming a granny was a journey of discovery, not just for me but also for my children. It was a delight to watch my sons turn into the fathers they'd always had in them – supportive, caring husbands and loving hands-on dads. I like to think they discovered me as the mother I had been to them.

I'm granny to 12 grandchildren, 10 girls and two boys and I was knocked sideways by the birth of my first grandchild, now a lovely woman of 27. I was ambushed by my emotions, I fell completely in love. I was besotted. But that wasn't the greatest thrill. I found

---

30   https://www.sunlife.co.uk/press-office/news/grandparents-childcare-salary/

through my grandchildren I could relive the emotions I thought I'd never feel again, a young mum feeling that all-consuming mother love I'd felt for my own children. And here it was, reborn, with my grandchildren.

My grandchildren have taught me a lot and so have my children and my children-in-law. I've written about being a granny and the lessons I learned. Over the years I found a few things that helped keep family relations sweet, and with an eye to maintaining good family relations, what a granny probably should and should not do. I even drew up a list of Golden Rules for Grandparents.

Of my grandchildren four are "my own" and eight are "step-grandchildren", a description I hate. I make no difference between them, they're all my grandchildren. Of course, when they're young, step-grandchildren don't know that there's no "blood tie" between us, all they know is the "love-tie" we have together and that I'm their granny. Mind you, these days with families being reframed by divorce and remarriage you might join a gaggle of grandparents. I'm one of four grannies in one family and the other three are higher ranking than I am. I'm conscious of my lowly status in the hierarchy. The grandchildren take no note of this and arrive at their own rankings. A lowly granny #3 or #4 to the adults could be a #1 to them. My eldest grandchild, the daughter of one of my stepsons and six years old at the time, gave me a note that brought tears to my eyes. It said "my best granny is Granny Miri". You may even find yourself being an extra granny. At a communal picnic, the small son of one of my daughter-in-law's girlfriends asked if Granny Miri could be his granny.

Of course, grandparenting isn't always plain sailing, it's not always happy families living together in perfect harmony. There's plenty of room for disagreement, differences of opinions, and tensions which, because of your wisdom, you're in a prime position to head off. One of the things I had to force myself to remember as a grandparent is you're not a parent, you're not the final arbiter of what's good for your grandchildren. I always had at the back of my mind that if things got really difficult, my children were in a position to prevent me from seeing my grandchildren. Winning an argument is never worth paying that price. I had no hesitation in backing off if it looked like relations were about to get strained. Remember, with your years of experience and wisdom, you're better placed than your children to be a conciliatory negotiator, the first to say sorry if you're wrong, to always ask how parents want things done, what their house rules are, and then do things their way even if you don't agree. I'll give you an example of this on the often tortured subject of baby sleep arrangements.

To set the scene, I was an adoring granny to a son's very young baby daughter and for the first three months I, my daughter-in-law and my son had got my granddaughter to sleep by nursing her till she dropped off and then placing her in her cot. She would cry sometimes for long periods, and we would again nurse her to sleep.

Then when she was about four months old, Ed said to me, "Mum, I don't like telling you what to do, but I'm going to tell you what to do. We've decided that the nightly sleep routine isn't good for the baby and it's not good for us, so we're going to change it. From now on we put her down in her cot, pat her back for a few moments and leave the room. If she cries, we wait a minute or two before going back into the room, we don't speak, we simply pat her on the back to reassure her that we're there and we leave the room again. I want you to repeat this routine until she's fallen asleep."

I confess it was agony sitting outside her room and listening to my granddaughter crying, but I obeyed their rules. And they were right to trust their baby daughter with a new sleep routine because after five days she'd learned what was expected of her and would hardly whimper when she was put into her cot. And it worked for me. There was no way I was going to throw a spanner in the works.

I swallowed hard and accepted that my son and my daughter-in-law had the right to decide how their baby should go to sleep. As a granny, you're perfectly placed to practise tolerance, flexibility and discretion and, in my case, to crawl over glass to keep communications open.

How to avoid tensions in your families

Try not to

… bear grudges even though it may be hard to forgive and forget. Life's too short. Overcome niggles and move on.

… harbour resentment, you won't be able to hide it and you'll become a granny who isn't nice to know, someone your family doesn't want to have around. You'll be less welcome than you would be if you suppressed your judgmental instincts.

… stand on ceremony. In the scheme of things, what does it cost you to give way? Just because you've lived a life, you don't necessarily know what's best for your grandchildren. But hard though it may be, you know when and how to exercise some restraint and back down.

… precipitate confrontation. Think about the future. You won't be easily forgiven and your children will always remember. Also, it's not easy for you to make amends for bad behaviour. Almost the greatest sin is to take sides between parents, especially if you're sticking up for your own son or daughter. Taking sides can be very upsetting. Favouritism could open up a rift that echoes down the years.

…get involved in a stalemate. There's no place for demanding respect in good grandparenting. Your children will see you as too difficult and you may not be invited back. When some of the most contentious baby issues come up like crying, feeding, bedtimes, weaning, toilet training, I think you have to hang back, go with parental preferences and keep a smile on your face.

Sex, Drugs & Walking Sticks

To my mind the self-effacing is worth it just to be in your grandchild's world, enjoying them, watching them grow up and being no more than a gentle guiding hand on their elbow.

One of the most positive things you can do for your children is to praise their efforts. I'm in no doubt there'll be lots of opportunities when you can praise them. In many ways, today's parents are a lot better than I was and it's as well to keep this at the back of your mind. I really do admire my children and stepchildren for the parents they are and for welcoming me into their families.

Does nature have a role for grandparents? Yes, it does. Women after the menopause used to just dwindle into old age but we have a very important role to play as grandparents in the scheme of things. And we share this role with several other animals, including elephants, whales and lions. Our role is to guide the mother, and to take care of her children so she's free to enlarge her family. In other words, grandmothers make it possible for younger women to have children. Other mammals, such as elephants, have matriarchal leaders who confer substantial benefits on the herd. I believe the human female is programmed to survive long after the menopause to support our children taking care of their children. Nonetheless, thinking you know best is a very dangerous step to take and something you should never assume. If you'd like to be a grandparent who's always welcome here are a few suggestions which, I've learned over the years, seem to work:

- Respect your children's boundaries (they can live their own lives).
- Never undermine your children or your grandchildren (you're their greatest fan).
- Praise your children on being good parents (every time you notice it).
- Keep communication open at all costs (be a conciliator).

- Offer support and advice without always expecting it to be accepted (you don't always know best).
- Visit only by invitation or mutual agreement (and take a small gift).
- Resist the temptation to get embroiled in emotional blackmail (stay at arm's length).
- Be a grandparent who's nice to know (rub along).
- Keep a well-developed sense of fairness and humour (smile a lot).
- Look for stories only you can tell (teach your grandchild about things you know, like your own childhood, gardening, travelling, knitting, sewing).

Outings grandparents can do with their grandchildren

There are lots of activities on offer for grandparents with their grandchildren so there's no need to feel at a loss for ideas.

- Music groups for babies from six months on are great fun and your grandchild can start learning to socialise.
- Baby massage classes, probably run by a health centre or local yoga teacher, can bring you very close to your grandchild.
- Swimming – once the baby is immunised ask at a local pool about parent-and-baby sessions. They'll welcome grandparents in the pool too.
- Find out if there's a baby-gym class in your area. Some leisure centres run these for babies as young as six months and their carers – you!
- Join in coffee mornings with parent-and-toddler groups.
- Baby movement classes may be run at leisure centres for babies from six months and can be bonding for your grandchild, and them with you.

H

Hair

HAIR IS SAID TO BE our crowning glory and I think it's good for us to think about it that way. With me, hair and how it looks is such an essential part of me that if my hair doesn't look good, I don't feel good. When I was doing television, I learned if I wasn't happy with my hair I wouldn't do a good show. It showed on the screen. I'm not proud of this, in fact, I'm rather ashamed. I should be more grown up. Our hair changes with age, it becomes thinner too, and bald patches may appear. Gone are the days of luxuriant tresses. If you suffer from an underactive thyroid it'll show in your hair which becomes sparse and falls out, and it may not regrow.

Another condition where there's frightening hair loss is after chemotherapy. It too will recover but it may take a few months.

Taking care of your hair (and your scalp)

This is the advice I used to give to patients in my clinic who had hair and scalp complaints.

- Never do anything to irritate your scalp when you're washing your hair, that only makes your scalp produce more grease. Instead, you should aim to "tranquilise" your scalp. So resist scrubbing. You'll also loosen hairs from the soft wet hair follicles and shed them.

- Never pull or tug on wet hair after washing. Wet hair stretches like elastic and easily breaks or tears. Use a detangler on your wet hair and a wide-toothed brush or comb.
- To avoid irritating your scalp don't brush or comb your hair too often or you'll boost your oil glands and your hair will look lank and dull.
- Restrict the use of use anti-dandruff shampoos to no more than once a fortnight. It'll keep your scalp happy as they contain ingredients such as selenium which is a scalp irritant. The scalp responds with more dandruff.
- There's no need to shampoo your hair twice, modern shampoos are very efficient so your hair needs only one wash. My recipe for gentle hair washing: mix two teaspoonfuls of baby shampoo in a glass of warm water and pour it over your already wet hair. Then massage the shampoo very gently into your hair. It's not necessary to scrub hard to work up a lather, just leave the shampoo on for about a minute and then rinse until the hair is clean. Always use a conditioner after hair washing to prevent tangling. After you've washed your hair, dab it dry with a towel rather than rubbing it vigorously.

I used a version of this recipe in my clinic. When I was a practising dermatologist and patients came to see me with a scalp or hair complaint, I would suggest they left all the glamorous shampoos on the shelf and instead used a carpet cleaner. Yes, a carpet cleaner. Why? Well, I and the other dermatologists knew that it was the most gentle shampoo you could find and there was good reason for this. The manufacturers of carpet cleaners have no desire to spoil your most treasured carpet so they make sure they're very gentle. Baby shampoo is also good.

I remember once being a guest on the Terry Wogan show and with me was the hairdressing king, Vidal Sassoon. When

I suggested that his clients should use carpet cleaner instead of his expensive shampoos Vidal became flustered and angry. Terry Wogan loved putting the two of us together and then watching the sparks fly. Mind you, I had science on my side, not to mention I was a trained dermatologist and understood the skin, scalp, and hair rather better than Mr Sassoon.

I have hypothyroidism (underactive thyroid) and over the years my hair has got thinner and thinner and I've relied more and more on hair pieces. Please don't reject hair pieces out of hand. Years ago I met a very glamorous actress with the most gorgeous thick hair. I really envied it. By the time I got to know her, she was wearing turbans.

"You have such beautiful hair", I said, "why do you hide it?"

"Oh, Miriam, that was all hair pieces!" She had used several at once. And so I was introduced to the world of hair pieces and have used them as needed to ginger up my hairstyle and they're good for morale. Later, I decided to go the whole hog. Throughout my life I'd always wanted long straight hair, and I realised a modern hairpiece could give me that with the minimum of bother. Upkeep is easy too. I take it off, wash it with a gentle shampoo, condition it and replace it. If I'm pressed, a hairdresser will come to the house to do it so it's convenient and not expensive when compared to weekly visits to the hairdressers' to keep my hair up to scratch. Hair pieces have given me enormous freedom and removed worries about thinning hair, bald patches. And I have no greys to cover up!

If you don't fancy a hair piece, consider buying a wig. There are plenty of cheap versions around and they're available at most hair salons, even in supermarkets. So give it a go and possibly discover a new you.

Thinning hair and bald patches can cause great heartache so I encourage you to think about camouflage. There are various different things you can try. Here are just a few.

Hair pieces

They come in all shapes and sizes, colours, and lengths. This is the safest and least painful way (in terms of health and money) to mask hair loss. You can choose to have them simply clipped into your own hair (very easy to remove) or semi-permanently attached to your own hair, either by tying, knotting or by being glued on to the scalp. The latter can stay firmly attached for about six weeks, when they're carefully taken off, washed, conditioned and re-applied. It's popular with men.

Hair weaving

As the name suggests, this weaves in replacement hair to existing hair to cover bald patches. The technique involves braiding strands of new hair onto the edges of the hair on your scalp. Weaving gives great results but it's high maintenance and must be cleaned carefully.

Coloured sprays

There are many in a range of shades to blend in with most hair colours. It's in the form of an organic dust and will cover bald patches if you spray it on several layers.

Men and baldness

Men are traditionally regarded as being less concerned than women about their hair now that there's a fashion for being bald, sported by glamorous stars and sportsmen. Nonetheless, most men feel thinning hair is ageing and can lead to loss of confidence and stress, so great even the most questionable remedies are sought after. Safe options for men are camouflage (see above), drugs and hair transplants. Minoxidil is such a drug and it was discovered by accident when it was being used in a clinical trial to treat high blood pressure. The researchers noticed that patients grew new scalp hair. So for once, a drug's side effects can be put to good use. Minoxidil works by boosting the blood supply to hair follicles, improving their nutrition so that hair starts growing again. It takes six months before the effects are visible. Once the treatment is finished, hair loss may start again. Minoxidil is not a permanent cure for baldness.

If you're after a permanent cure, hair transplants are always worth considering though the results can look "tufty", a bit like doll's hair if it's not done by a skilled and experienced practitioner. With transplants tiny strips of skin containing hairs are harvested from a donor site, usually at the back of the head. Small incisions are made in the recipient site with a punch, then the grafts are carefully inserted and a turban-like pressure dressing is applied. Reassuringly, hair transplants generally result in the permanent replacement of hair.

Remember your hair is dead. You can use moisturising conditioners and shampoos which make it "look" healthy but nothing more. The only live part of the hair is the growing root or follicle, deep in the skin and you can only get to that from the inside. The way to nourish your hair is to eat a good, healthy, balanced diet. Some women notice their hair is thinning after the menopause and this is because the female hormones oestrogen and progesterone fall precipitously. Hair follicles contain oestrogen receptors so hair growth may be kept healthy with HRT, though this shouldn't ever be the sole reason for taking HRT.

Health Checks – Essential

IT'S WISE TO KEEP A record of your health checks in a special diary noting the name of the health check, where you have it done and who does it for you. In this way you can provide a kind of timetable for yourself. Transfer it to your diary, or put the annual timetable somewhere in your kitchen where you'll see it all the time and therefore not forget a particular check.

Here are some suggestions as to how often you might arrange those checks.

- Visit your dentist **every six months** to check up on the health of your teeth and your gums.
- An eye check from either an ophthalmologist, an eye doctor, or an optician **every year.**
- Have your ears examined by your doctor **every two years.**
- Your blood pressure should be checked **every two years** and by yourself at home, say **monthly**, with a simple blood pressure device from Boots including a pamphlet on how to use it.
- If you've ever been a smoker or are still smoking, you should have a chest X-ray **once a year** arranged by your GP.
- If it's appropriate, a mammogram, a cervical smear and a PSA **every three years.**
- **Every five years** you should have a physical examination by a doctor, an ovarian ultrasound, a sigmoidoscopy which looks directly at the large bowel and stool testing for blood, arranged by your GP.
- Check your blood cholesterol **once a year.**

Heartburn

MOST PEOPLE HAVE HAD HEARTBURN usually following a large, rich meal. As the name implies, you feel a burning sensation behind your breastbone, which may sometimes go right up to your throat. Most of us gain relief from sucking an antacid tablet which neutralises the acid in the stomach and takes away the stinging sensation of heartburn.

The cause is often a hiatus hernia, more common as we get older as the stomach and gullet become slack and stretchy. What happens is the opening in the diaphragm, through which the gullet (oesophagus) passes from the chest into the stomach below, gets bigger and a small part of the stomach can slip back up into the chest. That allows regurgitation of the acid contents of the stomach into the gullet where they cause inflammation, soreness and eventually ulceration. It's unwise to ignore these symptoms and pass them off simply as "a bit of indigestion". Heartburn is much more serious than indigestion.

Hiatus hernia is often called GORD, gastro-oesophageal reflux disease. It doesn't go away on its own therefore once it's occurred you'll have it for years depending on how old you are. The seven million Brits who have it should not ignore it. Occasional heartburn isn't dangerous as cells at the bottom of the gullet which are burned by the stomach acid can heal themselves. However, heartburn over the long-term is dangerous. Persistent reflux can injure the cells to the extent they develop a condition called Barrett's oesophagus, and that's precancerous. In other words, there's a risk they can become cancerous if not treated.

The number of patients who develop Barrett's oesophagus is about one in 300 a year but if cancer develops it's a very aggressive cancer. Less than one in six patients survive for more than five years. So if you have long-term heartburn it's imperative you see your doctor who can arrange for tests to diagnose Barrett's oesophagus and stop cancer taking over.

Treatment used to remove about two thirds of the gullet but this has been superseded by a new treatment which is so simple it can be done as an outpatient. It burns away the precancerous or cancerous tissues using a fine electric needle, taking only about 20 minutes. Afterwards, new healthy cells can grow back. This simple procedure, pioneered by University College Hospital in London, gives long-lasting protection against oesophageal cancer. I'd like to tell you how the diagnosis of Barret's oesophagus is made because it's another ingenious English discovery. It's called the "capsule sponge test". All you do is swallow a pill on a string. It dissolves in the stomach and releases a sponge to which cells cling as the sponge is removed by pulling on the string. This test is sensitive enough to detect changes in oesophageal cells much earlier than before, so cancer is detected sooner. The results are usually excellent. Get in touch with Cancer Research UK if you'd like to find out more about it.

There are ways to lower your risk of getting cancer of the oesophagus. If you're a smoker the sooner you quit the better because people who smoke, and those who drink alcohol, have an increased risk of oesophageal cancer. It's wise to cut down on your drinking. Your diet is important (for all cancers). So eating plenty of fruit and vegetables may help to reduce your risk. You should aim for five portions a day and choose a variety of different coloured fruits and vegetables (yellow, orange, dark red) so that you get a broad range of vitamins and minerals.

Here are more ways you can help yourself...

- At night in bed, don't lie down, especially if you have a full stomach. Besides raising the head of your bed (on a couple of books), sleep with two or three pillows so that you're at an angle of 45 degrees.
- Try to avoid foods which worsen acid reflux, such as fatty foods, fizzy drinks, alcohol and coffee.
- Being overweight makes hiatus hernia worse, so lose a bit if you can.

- Reduce the size of your meals, especially those you eat late in the evening, it's better to eat little and often.
- Avoid bending.

High Heels

HIGH HEELS PLAY HAVOC WITH your back because they thrust your trunk forward and your back muscles have to compensate. They're also bad for your feet so fortunately for us the fashion for high heels has come full circle. Comfort is all, and we're back to flats and trainers. Anyone of my generation will remember the slavery to high heels. From my teens onwards, I wore vertiginously high heels. Long before Sarah Jessica Parker and *Sex & The City*, I was addicted to Manolo Blahnik and Jimmy Choo until my back gave out and I was forced into lower heels.

We willingly suffered the discomfort, corns, bunions and crushed toes. I remember speaking to a PR exec to whom high heels were a badge of office, meaning dizzyingly high Prada heels. I asked her if they were comfortable.

"Heavens no", she said, "I take a couple of paracetamol before I wear them so my feet don't feel the pain. Even so, I wear them only for a few hours."

So, at about the age of 65, when walking became the only exercise I could take regularly, I literally threw away all my heels and settled for flats. In trainers I was free to walk whenever and wherever the opportunity presented itself. The revolution was just beginning and professional women were daring to wear trainers to work. Seems such a small thing now but then it was part of a feminist revolution. Not quite bra burning but another nail in the coffin of women having to conform.

As we get older it's necessary we free ourselves from what fashion dictates so don't hesitate to get rid of your high heels, be more comfortable and always ready for a stroll.

Protecting your feet from the effects of ageing

General health

Being overweight adds to the pressure on your feet so keep checking your weight. Get your feet examined regularly if you have diabetes, peripheral arterial disease, problems with the nerves in your feet (peripheral neuropathy), foot deformity or deformities of the toenails.

Skin care

Check out your feet every day. Attend to any breaks or cracks in the skin. Remove hard skin with a pumice stone. Trim and file your toenails straight across to help prevent ingrown toenails. Moisturise your feet to prevent calluses and cracks.

Exercise

Regular walking is great for the circulation in your feet and helps prevent swelling. Ankle circling is excellent as is raising yourself onto your toes and back down onto your heels several times while holding onto something to keep you steady. It's not good to sit for long periods with your feet hanging down. If moving around is difficult for you, sit with your feet elevated.

Shoes

It's best if you avoid high heels and pointed toes altogether. Opt for those which support your feet like lace-up shoes. Shoes with an ankle strap and shoes that hold your heel firm give the best support. Far and away the best support shoe is trainers, especially if you choose a sports trainer that will support your arch and hold your heel firmly in line. My favourite are Asics. Make sure that your shoes are big enough if your feet have a tendency to swell. Your footwear should be comfortable and warm.

Hormones

A HORMONE IS A CHEMICAL MESSENGER that's produced in one part of the body, enters the bloodstream, circulates around the body and has an effect on a distant organ. So, for instance, testosterone is produced in the testes, circulates around the body and has effects on hair growth on the head, the face, armpits, and pubic area. It gives men their muscular shape and importantly, their sexuality, including sex drive, libido, and erections. Sperm are under its control too.

In women, oestrogen is produced in the ovary and has early effects on forming the breasts, the growth of pubic hair and body odours in the armpits and pubic area. It, along with the second powerful female hormone, progesterone, result in menstruation, periods, with monthly bleeding from the womb, uterus. It's essential to keep a pregnancy going too.

A word about the female hormones oestrogen and progesterone

Two hormones dominate a girl and a woman's life, oestrogen and progesterone. Having done quite a lot of hormone research, I always think of oestrogen as being the nice, friendly one and progesterone as being something of an impatient bully. These two hormones are crucial to a woman's developing fertility. They're produced by the ovaries with small contributions from the adrenal glands and most importantly from fat cells. Singly and together, they're extremely powerful, being responsible for puberty, the menstrual cycle, pregnancy, and when withdrawn, the menopause. Oestradiol is the main oestrogen in a woman's body, it's produced in the ovaries for the whole of her fertile life. Good news. It's possible to boost your oestrogen levels naturally. My favourite way is exercise. During exercise a male hormone (dehydroepiandrosterone) which is made in the adrenal glands, is converted to oestrogen. It's only in small amounts, but it's oestrogen nonetheless. The more you exercise, the more you'll flood your body with oestrogen. Vitamin B also helps your body to create and use oestrogen.

Oestrogen and progesterone affect many, if not all, of the organs in a woman's body and they contribute to body weight, to hair growth and to bone and muscle strength. Oestrogen is the hormone of the first part of the menstrual cycle and when I was in my 40s and suffering from PMS every month, the only really happy time I had during the month was when I was under the influence of oestrogen. And the sensation of oestrogen rising. This happens as your period ends and, as I felt my oestrogen levels rising, it was the most pleasurable part of the month by a long chalk.

Progesterone puts in an appearance in the week after ovulation (at the start of the third week of the month) and it's not necessarily good news for us, because progesterone is a close relative of testosterone. In other words progesterone can make you impatient, bad tempered, and totally unreasonable. When I found myself under the influence of this unforgiving hormone I felt, at my worst moments, I could kill anyone, including myself. It can be a depressing hormone.

Progesterone, the "pregnancy hormone" and the major hormone of the second half of the menstrual cycle is important for menstruation and, surprisingly, sperm production. Yes, men have some too. The ovaries produce it as well as the placenta, and the adrenal glands that lie on top of the kidneys. During menstruation, it prepares the uterus for the advent of a pregnancy so progesterone thickens the lining of the uterus, ready for implantation and it supports the early development of the unborn baby. The upside of progesterone is that, in pregnancy, it helps to *lower* anxiety and mood swings. It acts as a tranquiliser and as a natural antidepressant. It may even help in postpartum depression.

You can imagine what happens to your body and brain when two such crucial hormones plummet. Catastrophe. Menopause.

There are of course, other hormones in the body such as thyroid hormone, insulin, and neurotransmitters produced in the brain such as serotonin and dopamine but none as dominant in women as oestrogen and progesterone.

Testosterone in ageing

Testosterone, primarily a male sex hormone, is also present in women and partly responsible for their libido. In men it controls the physical and sexual development of young men, being responsible for the growth of the penis and secondary sexual characteristics such as the voice-breaking and the masculine shape, broad shoulders and narrow waist. It propels the development of the testes and prostate gland. Its most important function, however, is sperm production, sperm quality and sperm numbers. Testosterone gives men a sense of well-being, and helps to produce red blood cells in the bone marrow. It's also responsible for aggression and violence.

I found this out for myself when I was writing a book about sex and I was mentioning that testosterone supplements were sometimes given to menopausal women to boost sex drive. I thought to myself, I can't write about testosterone without having experienced it myself and so I took some testosterone for three or four days, after which I was compelled to stop. Why? I've never felt so aggressive, bad tempered, impatient, argumentative, and angry as I did while I was on testosterone. I felt I'd looked through a window at what men are feeling all the time. Only I was able to turn my testosterone off and they aren't. Women do have small quantities of testosterone in their bodies. It's produced in the adrenal glands and contributes to our assertiveness and muscle strength as well as libido.

As older age approaches, men begin to wonder if they have enough testosterone, and it's true, levels do tend to drop from the age of about 30-40, but it's a gentle slide down. Men don't go through a male menopause like women. The menopause is the sudden withdrawal of female sex hormones in women with the resultant shock to the system with symptoms of hot flushes, night sweats and dry vagina. Men experience nothing like this sudden drop.

Not many doctors subscribe to the idea of giving men supplementation for a few signs of low testosterone. In middle age onwards testosterone is linked to heart disease. Most men will eventually feel the effects of a dropping testosterone level and here's how:

- Putting on weight around the waist, a beer belly.
- Muscles diminish in size, and are no longer as strong as they were.
- Problems getting off to sleep and staying asleep.
- You won't be aware of it, but your bone density is being eroded.
- Your sex drive is not what it was.
- Difficulty getting and maintaining an erection, ED, and your sperm count is lower than in your prime.
- There's always Viagra, and penile injections that will give you an erection lasting an hour or so. Worth a try if you're healthy. Speak to your doctor as you may need a heart check before taking Viagra and similar drugs.

If you feel that you'd like to try testosterone supplements it's not always plain sailing. Testosterone therapy may worsen sleep apnoea where your breathing stops and starts while you're asleep. It may affect your heart. Testosterone replacement therapy (TRT) is rarely considered until lifestyle changes and other medical interventions have been tried.

Intravaginal HRT

I've been mentioning HRT in various places in my book and it strikes me that I should say a few words about HRT, in older women.

I took HRT, latterly in gel form smoothed on my skin, until I was 63 years old. This is too old. I should have stopped before but to be honest I didn't want to lose the edge that I felt HRT gave me. Before I stopped I thought stopping would be like falling off a cliff. It wasn't of course.

In general it's thought that women should take HRT for menopausal symptoms for about five or six years max if they're suitable subjects. After that side effects might occur. By the time I came off HRT I had been on it for 12 years, a length of time considered too long by the majority of doctors.

For women over 60 I think the only situations where HRT, in the form of oestrogen, could be legitimately used would be a dry, sore vagina and repeated urinary tract infections. The oestrogen is given in a special way, intravaginally, either as a cream or a tiny pellet which is introduced with an applicator. Speak to your doctor about it if you have soreness in and around your vagina, and if you're having repeated attacks of cystitis. Symptoms from a dry vagina will be relieved by intravaginal oestrogen too.

Hypothermia

WE ASSOCIATE HYPOTHERMIA (low body temperature) with old people living in rooms without heating but in fact healthy young men who are exposed to cold for a long time at very low temperatures will also suffer hypothermia. It's always serious due to a fall in body core temperature. This means many of the vital organs such as the heart, lungs, kidneys, liver and the brain gradually cease to work. Our bodies are designed to work optimally when our temperature is around 37°C (98.6F) and an awful lot of bodily functions stop working at temperatures much lower than that. However, in hypothermia, temperatures have been recorded as low as 21°C (78.5F).

An old person just sitting still in a chair and not moving about may suffer a drop in body temperature in cold weather and where there's little heating. Most of us keep our core temperature up in the normal range by moving around in cold weather. Muscle activity produces heat and helps to maintain a normal body temperature. A drop in temperature doesn't have to be great, a small drop of only a few degrees in an old, immobile person can be very serious. The signs you should be aware of are slow or slurred speech, a slow pulse, confusion and sleepiness but no shivering. A straightforward test for hypothermia is to feel those parts of the body which are normally warm, like the inside of the thighs or the abdomen. If these places are cold, it's an emergency and you must get medical help.

The treatment is to raise body temperature. In older people re-warming should be slow in order to avoid any harm. Warming up old people too quickly is dangerous and they may die suddenly as a result. Warming up should be carefully controlled and not be any greater than one degree per hour. No direct heat should be applied.

Of course, ideally, no old person should be living in accommodation where the temperature might go so low they suffer hypothermia. Equally, no older person should live on their own without a family member or a friend visiting them regularly to make sure their accommodation is warm, they have plenty of warm clothing, and eat hot food regularly. If a person's temperature drops below 32°C then they should be rushed to hospital. Above 32°C it would be possible to treat the person at home, but be sure and ask your doctor for advice, and follow it.

Here are a few things you can do to keep yourself warm around the house:

- Maintain a temperature of 18°C in your home, if at all possible.
- If you feel the cold wear several layers (or a fluffy onesie).
- Cover all your extremities with hat, gloves, socks.
- A hot water bottle or a heat pad can keep your core warm if you hug it.
- Warm your bed up with a hot water bottle before getting into it.
- Stand up every half an hour and walk around a bit.

While hypothermia may occur when someone falls in a cold place and can't move, we now know that it can occur in quite different circumstances with some serious illnesses such as a heart attack, a stroke and with some medicines. In fact, instead of a raised temperature the body temperature goes down, possibly due to medical shock, low blood pressure and a cold, clammy skin.

I

IBS

IBS IS COMMON, IT CAN interfere with everyday life, and it's chronic, so it may start when you're in your 50s or 60s, but it could linger for longer.

The symptoms you may suffer are many and varied, including abdominal cramps, diarrhoea, constipation, bloating due to gas build-up, nausea, an urgent call to stool, tiredness and backache. The actual cause is unknown, and it's described as "functional" as there's no visible damage to the gastrointestinal tract, GIT. This distinguishes it from inflammatory bowel disease, a completely different condition where there's always inflammation of the bowel lining.

Symptoms of IBS can vary in frequency and severity. Some attacks may last days, weeks, even months.

Many reasons have been put forward as the cause of IBS including food sensitivity, gut sensitivity, stress, anxiety, and family history – it's possible that there's a genetic connection.

Remedies may or may not work, but the mainstays of treatment are lifestyle changes and some medicines, the major lifestyle change being attention to diet. Trigger foods if they're known should be avoided and there's research showing the FODMAP (Fermentable Oligosaccharides, Disaccharides, Monosaccharides, and Polyols) exclusion diet does work for about eight out of ten people[31] because it reduces fermentation and gas in the bowel. So consult your doctor about it. To my mind bowel oversensitivity is the root of the problem in the way that in irritable bladder syndrome, the bladder is oversensitive to the presence of urine and urges you to empty it.

Hydration is always important, so you should sip water at regular intervals through the day. Regular exercise helps, as does enough sleep. It'll help if you get some control over the stress in your life by learning about stress management. Your doctor can give you medications to treat the diarrhoea and constipation. In the main, IBS is a lifelong condition but the good news is that it's manageable with lifestyle changes and some medication.

Incontinence

HOW TIMES HAVE CHANGED! I can remember as recently as the 80s, incontinence was never mentioned. It was too embarrassing a subject to air. Quite often people with incontinence were so embarrassed they were even reluctant to mention the word to a doctor. A far cry from today where women and TV ads confess to incontinence and even talk about "my bulky pee pants". And it's right that we should be open and candid about a condition that around 40% of people in the older age group suffer from.

While we tend to focus on leaks from the bladder and we think of incontinence as purely down to bladder weakness, I've always thought it's due partly to "brain" incontinence. That's why incontinence is made worse by anxiety, stress and being in a strange environment like a hospital or care home. Being mobile is important

---

31   https://www.hopkinsmedicine.org/health/wellness-and-prevention/fodmap-diet-what-you-need-to-know

too as many older people have difficulty getting to the loo quickly enough and worry about not being able to hold on. That worry can precipitate leakage.

Stress incontinence (leaking with coughing, heavy lifting) of women in their late 40s and 50s is generally due to damage to the pelvic floor muscles while giving birth. But we see incontinence more and more often as we grow older as tissues thin, weaken and stretch.

Incontinence affecting people in their late 60s and 70s may be due to something as simple as a change from familiar surroundings. It may also start during any acute illness and will disappear when the illness is cured. Oversensitivity and overactivity of the bladder may result from a stroke and some water tablets may make incontinence worse. As you get older think about adapting the lavatory to your needs by moving it to an easier position. You'll be helped by going to the loo every two hours whether you feel the urge or not.

In men, incontinence is quite often due to benign prostatic enlargement, BPH. Surgical treatment is an option to relieve it. An internal cutting knife passed up a fine tube inside the urethra so that excess prostate tissue can be shaved away and the passage opened up.

There's a large menu of incontinence aids for both women and men, focussing on individual needs and preferences. Age and both physical and mental conditions should be taken into account. Pants should be soft, light, open, stretchy, designed to fit any person. Knickers should have wide legs. If a dress is worn it helps if there are flaps at the back which can be moved out of the way easily. A waterproof bed sheet avoids embarrassing wet beds.

At any age and in both women and men, exercising your pelvic floor muscles which support the bladder, will help your incontinence.

Pelvic floor exercises, for men too

These exercises are like an insurance policy for the rest of your life, for both women and men. So practise pelvic floor exercises till they become second nature and you'll have fewer problems with incontinence and vaginal prolapse. They can also improve sexual enjoyment. Here's a well-tried routine.

- Pull up the muscles "down below" for five seconds, then let them go for five seconds, then pull them up again. Your pelvic floor muscles grow stronger with every exercise till you can pull them up with ease.
- As quickly as possible, tighten and relax the muscles ten times, as though they're "fluttering".
- The last phase is to bear down, as if you were emptying your bowels, more at the front than at the back and hold for five seconds. As your pelvic floor gets stronger, increase to ten contractions ten times a day. You'll soon find you can exercise your pelvic floor anywhere, any time, even sitting down, walking and in bed.

Inheritance

WHETHER YOU HAVE A LOT to leave your family or very little, it's worth starting those difficult conversations about your death and what your family will inherit from you. You can do this with a close friend or with the solicitor if you wish. I firmly believe you should also discuss with the beneficiaries of inheritance what they'll inherit from you.

Most people worry about inheritance tax (IHT) which covers

property, money and possessions. There will be none to pay if your estate is valued at less than £350,000 or leave all of it to a spouse, a civil partner, a charity, or a community amateur sports club. But even if no inheritance taxes are due you may still have to report the value. If you give away your home to your children, whether they're adopted, fostered or stepchildren, the threshold rises to £500,000 before you qualify for IHT. IHT is charged at a rate of 40% on the value of your estate above the threshold and it's reduced if you leave more than 10% to charity on a pro rata basis. There is also "taper relief" on gifts that you have given in the seven years preceding your death based on a pro rata reduction for every year out of the seven you have lived since you passed on the gift. The payment of any IHT should come from the funds of your estate and are paid to the tax authority, HMRC. IHT on gifts only accrues if you give away more than £350,000 and die within seven years.

I always thought it was morbid to make a will. In the event it's far from it. What a will does is to make you examine all your assets and decide how you'll dispose of them. And that brings a sense of having closed the circle and taken care of the family and friends who are dear to you. The legal side of things can be daunting but you just need a good solicitor. I have found the best way to choose one is with a recommendation from family or friends. Then it becomes not an obstacle but a fulfilling way to be remembered after you've gone. Before seeking advice from a solicitor establish what their costs are and decide if you can afford them. Also you can contact Citizens Advice, plus many charities will provide you with a free service.

J

Joy

I'VE HAD MORE JOY IN my life than anyone has the right to expect. Happiness as well, though happiness is fleeting and joy is not. Joy is almost a way of life, and for me it's close to optimism. My mum used to face adversity with one of her many adages, "every cloud has a silver lining", and if you're on the lookout for silver linings, there are quite a few of them about waiting to be discovered. There's the instant delight that comes from recognising something wonderful and can be felt through our senses – sight, sound, taste, touch. But for me, the source of greatest joy resides in people and, in particular, my children and grandchildren. And it is pleasure, but infinite pleasure. The kind that can't be put into words because it springs from such a deep part of the brain it's inexpressible. Much of my joy comes to me through love, especially unsolicited love like a spontaneous act of kindness. It's tangible, like a taste in the mouth.

The hallmark of joy is intensity, you feel it with your whole being. Joy is clearly good for you because it brings long-lasting contentment with life and imbues you with hope. I think joy is a state of mind, a state where we seek joy, feel joy, accept joy, not from external events, but from the readiness inside of us to find it. When I'm joyful, I do feel a sense of wholeness and completeness, a sense of infinite possibilities.

I remember once playing with my children in the garden and I felt joy so intense, in my children, in my life, in my husband, in my work that I honestly thought, "I have everything life has to offer. I can gladly die now".

There's a bit of science to joy. It's thought to be down to neurotransmitters in the brain. These are chemicals released in the brain and are responsible for a lot of our good feelings. When I find myself "in flow" which by definition is when you're fully immersed in a difficult task, you're fully focussed, fully involved, feeling high on your ability to match the job – that's a kind of joy too. It's a perfect balance between what's required of you and what you can do. Well, when I'm in flow I can feel great joy just from my brain working. All my life I've felt joy when I'm learning. Even as a child I felt just finding out about something was a reliable source of joy, achievement less so. Feeling joy does us good. It's good for the heart and it teaches us resilience.

Joy seems to me mystical because I don't know where it comes from and I don't know how I'm feeling it. It's intangible and it fills me up completely. Fills me up with hope. I find myself breathing deeply. I'm certain that gratitude is part of joy and when we feel joy in that sense, the emotion is so deep it quite often brings us to tears. Joy always has an element of spirituality. If you think of joy at its most extreme like rapture and bliss, we recognise that joy is a kind of pinnacle of feeling. We even talk about "being on cloud nine" and "being on top of the world".

And now for those neurotransmitters. Is joy simply a flooding of the brain with feel-good hormones like dopamine, serotonin, endorphins and oxytocin, neurotransmitters we hear quite a lot about? Dopamine is the reward neurotransmitter and makes us feel good about ourselves. Serotonin affects our mood and makes us calm and optimistic. Endorphins are secreted by the body during exercise and when we suffer pain. They're our natural opioids and relieve pain, but they can also make us feel euphoric, high. Oxytocin reaches very high levels during and after childbirth (it's thought to be responsible for a woman's mother love) and is rightly called the love hormone or the cuddle hormone because it's released during bonding and intimacy. It makes us feel we can trust, through a loving connection. Most of all it makes us feel love.

I can hear you saying, "Well, that's all well and good but I've never felt anything like that and to be honest, I don't know how to feel joy." Yes, I accept that and it's set me thinking. I think the easiest route to feeling joy is to plumb your deepest emotions and give them space, let them envelope you. Give them free rein. Don't try to submerge them. And then open your eyes and see what's around you. Use that joy to wonder at the beauty around you and if it isn't immediate, go somewhere like a park and wonder at nature.

What I feel when I'm joyful is spiritual. It fills me with wonder. It's enriching, nourishing, thrilling, blissful. I'm grateful I've had so much of it in my life.

K

K – Potassium

THE CHEMICAL SYMBOL FOR POTASSIUM is a simple K and I'm including it because it's a vital mineral in the body. It participates in regulating your fluid balance. It's very important for good nerve and muscle function, and for controlling blood pressure. It allows the nerves to respond to stimulation and muscles to contract (tighten) including the muscles of the heart. It's particularly important to the heart because it helps the heart maintain the electrical signals necessary for a regular heartbeat. It supports muscle contractions and helps to move nutrients into, and waste products out of, cells. Potassium tends to keep the blood pressure low to normal and therefore counteracts the effect of sodium on blood pressure.

People with low potassium may notice muscle weakness, muscle cramps and possibly an abnormal heart rhythm like palpitations. A crucial sign of potassium deficiency is a high blood pressure and thereby hangs a tale. I'd been to see a doctor for a heart check-up and he took a blood sample for analysis. A few days later I got a call from him out of the blue when he said, "Miriam, get in a taxi and come to hospital immediately because your potassium levels are exceedingly low." And indeed when I got into hospital they were very low and my blood pressure was consequently sky high. It was resistant to the usual treatments for bringing blood pressure down. We decided my very high blood pressure, resistant to treatment, was due to my very low potassium.

But how did my potassium get so low? An endocrinologist was called in to see if I had any endocrine abnormalities which might have caused the low potassium. None was found. And then one day a rather old and very experienced endocrinologist visited me saying, "I want to get to the bottom of why your potassium is so low." And he asked me if I had, by any chance, been eating liquorice. You know that delicious soft, black liquorice. Well, I had. I love soft chewable black liquorice and always had a bag in the house and dipped into it almost every day. "That, he said, is the culprit." Liquorice depletes the body of potassium and as soon as I stopped eating it my potassium levels started to rise and my blood pressure started to fall.

Within a week to 10 days of liquorice abstinence my blood pressure was within the normal range. I'm sure it would be okay to eat the odd bit of liquorice but felt it was better to go cold turkey so I haven't had any since that dramatic incident. In general, it's pretty easy to keep your potassium levels normal. Just eat foods that are high in potassium such as bananas, avocados, sweet potatoes, leafy greens like spinach, dried fruits and tomatoes. You can further boost your potassium intake by eating broccoli, yoghurt, salmon and lentils.

L

—

Living Will

YOU MAY HAVE HEARD ABOUT a living will and wondered what it's for. It's to make sure the doctors who are caring for you comply with your wishes and refrain from subjecting you to any medical interventions or treatment aimed at prolonging your life beyond a certain point if you don't wish it. It's known as an Advance Directive where you can set out on a form any treatments you don't want, even if you're seriously ill and unable to tell doctors what you want to happen to you. If you want to make sure that you're not given, for example, life-prolonging treatment when you suffer a serious heart attack, your living will makes sure your wishes are honoured. A living will is really the opportunity for you to take charge of your treatment in the latter stages of your life. It makes sure you're not kept alive when ordinarily you wouldn't want to be, for instance, being kept alive indefinitely on a life support machine.

A living will is not only for you to decide how much medical intervention you want at the end of your life, it's also for your friends and family who'll be looking after you to help them to make difficult decisions about your treatment. You could, for instance, have terminal damage to your brain due to a stroke, injury, dementia or motor neurone disease and if your family doesn't know what your preferences are, doctors may keep you on a life support machine, or in a deep coma being fed through a tube or intravenously. In this kind of situation all your bodily functions are under the control of machines to keep you alive. I know I don't want to go through any such extreme treatment to keep me alive so I've completed a living will for the peace of mind of my family.

Your living will isn't set in tablets of stone. You can add to it, amend it so it fits with your preferences as you get older. On the form there's a section where you can record your beliefs, your religion, and thoughts about death. The British Medical Association, the Royal College of Nursing and the Government have all confirmed they support living wills, which brings us into line with the living will all patients who enter a US hospital have to complete before treatment is started.

You may ask if a living will is legal and binding? Well, it is if the following conditions are met:

- You're over the age of 18 when you make the will.
- You're not suffering from any mental distress and you're mentally able.
- At the time you made your living will you were fully informed about how it works and its consequences.
- The living will takes account of all the situations or circumstances which may arise in your later life.
- In making the decision, you haven't been pressured or influenced by anyone else.
- You have not made any statements or performed any actions that would contradict your living will wishes. Though it makes good sense to read it through, reconsider and reconfirm it every few years, updating it with the date and your signature. If necessary, speak to a doctor to see if everything you have asked for can be taken care of. It would be wise to send your GP a copy of your living will.

- You have got to the stage of being mentally incapable of making any medical decision because you're unconscious or otherwise unfit.

If you're thinking about making a living will but don't know how to start, the website of the charity Compassion in Dying can help you (https://compassionindying.org.uk/). You don't need a solicitor to make a living will.

The charity suggests you:

1. Fill in the form (you can find their online template) here: https://www.advancedecision.service.compassionindying.org.uk/ or you can print out a paper copy if you prefer.
2. Print, sign and get it witnessed (the witness can be anyone, including a relative).
3. Share a copy (with your relatives, GP, local hospital and local ambulance trust).
4. Review it regularly (every two years or sooner if your health or wishes change).

Loneliness

IT'S AT LEAST A DECADE since I began to think of loneliness as an illness, instead of just being something that happened to people who live alone and was worse in old age. Since then, we've discovered many consequences of loneliness which can be considered serious diseases. Loneliness, whenever we come across it, has to be taken seriously. It takes its toll on anyone, even a young person, but it's particularly detrimental to older people where living alone can become dangerous. Boredom can quickly turn into anger, then descend into apathy and finally into stagnation. Almost without realising it, alertness and engagement falter and then the loss of a grip on mental and physical skills inevitably follows.

Becoming a widow several years ago didn't make me feel lonely, it made me feel apathetic. Looking back, I realise I'd completely lost the taste for life. That was my way of grieving. So I shunned the usual advice that's recommended to newly widowed people like staying in touch with friends, going out and about to the cinema, theatre or opera, joining in parties. I had no relish for any of that but I did do something that I think resulted in my looking after my mental wellbeing when I was alone. I indulged myself. I did things which I love and require little effort – and a degree of selfishness. I read a newspaper from cover to cover every day, something I've never done before but love. I listened to music all the time, I read books continuously, and I stayed very close to family, particularly to my grandchildren, and over a year or so my apathy gradually waned.

A prominent feature of loneliness is isolation; isolation from not just people of our own age, but also isolation from young people whose interests, even their language, and their attachment to social media are alien. Bereavement is very tough on older people when they lose someone with whom they had a close emotional relationship. When isolation descends into desolation, feeling alone, and forgotten we may feel emotionally forsaken, similar to someone in solitary confinement. We all need an outlet for our emotional needs and instincts whatever our age but physical frailty makes loneliness worse. We're living longer, particularly women, and this longevity means more older women than men are left alone and isolated. Loneliness for many people translates into more than being alone, it means loss of loving emotional ties.

The most lonely I've ever felt was in my 50s during a media tour in America for one of my books. During the week I was shunted between interviews by a PR but at weekends I was left to my own devices. Once, in Arizona I was stuck in a hotel in the desert and when I left the hotel for a walk a police car drew alongside me. The officer accused me of vagrancy and I had to take him to my hotel and show him my return air ticket. I tried taking a taxi to a shopping mall just to see people. It was soul-destroying and back in the hotel I listened to music on my Walkman in an attempt to ease the desolation I was feeling. As soon as I knew the UK was awake (the UK was eight hours ahead of me in Arizona) I phoned home. It was then that I realised loneliness isn't just about being alone, nor is it about being with people who love you. It's about being without people *you* love. Being unable to *give* love.

Families can do a lot to relieve this loneliness and isolation by keeping an eye on an elderly relative, if necessary by rota, to form a supportive network of family and friends and to provide the emotional contact everyone longs for.

Here are some of my thoughts on how best to tackle loneliness

Keep up strong friendships if you can

Friendships are so nourishing to us. They're precious, counteract loneliness and help protect our mental health. They may even lengthen life.

Don't neglect yourself while looking after others

Many of us feel we have to look after others but the stress and strain of caregiving can take quite a toll on your own health and lead to your becoming isolated from the outside world. It's important to find ways to care for your own health while caring for others.

Be active together
> One of the best ways of keeping up connections is to do physical activities with other people you know, like the local gym can have a positive effect on your health and who knows, you may connect with new friends.

Build relationships
> Long-term relationships are important throughout your life but especially as you get older because they make you feel connected and can improve your mental and physical well-being.

Spend time with your grandkids
> It's worth staying fit just to be with your grandchildren. The strong emotional bonds between you and your grandkids can help children learn how to deal with their own feelings and behaviours, and you with yours.

Managing loneliness

Keep a diary
> You can use loneliness as a spur to help you as long as you face up to it. When my husband died I found keeping a diary opened my eyes. I wrote down the times when I felt most bereft, and got a clearer picture of my sad times. In doing so, I got them into perspective. They seemed less consuming and became less frequent.

Recognise your feelings
> If you miss the physical closeness of a cuddle, a hug, holding hands, and missing sex, acknowledge it. As a widow myself I recognise that now and then I'd like some male company and just being looked after by a caring man. But I find I'm reluctant to make a move. It's normal to dither about joining the dating game.

I doubt I ever shall. Like many bereaved and widowed women I find I like being alone, single, and mistress of my own destiny.

Split up your time

Planning your time can go a long way to overcoming feelings of loneliness. Even if you don't want to follow a timetable, a bit of planning will give you a new point of view about possibilities, particularly if you think about filling days with different activities.

So you could take up a new hobby or learn a new language at night school. One evening you could have some friends around to yours and on another visit them. Find out what's on at the local cinema, theatre or concert hall and arrange to go with a grandchild or a friend. I go to the cinema with one granddaughter who loves films. Take care of your fitness with pilates, yoga classes, or work out in the gym.

Don't forget home hobbies like gardening, carpentry, and doing a bit of painting and decorating around the house. Make space on Saturday nights for something special like a local club where you find people interested in the same things as you. Don't turn your nose up at a singles club, dancing club, the local golf club, and a bridge club which run celebratory Saturday nights. Spend a lot of time planning Sundays because they can be long days. To my mind the best way of spending Sundays is to have friends or family for a casual lunch or brunch when people can come and go. If you don't want to cook, ask each of your guests to bring a dish around.

Don't stay at home alone

Whatever your age, I'm a great fan of "getting out of the house". It's such a mood booster. Just seeing people in the street (and smiling if you can) can change the complexion of a day. If you're near open spaces or a park, practise some mindfulness and notice dogs, flowers, birds and trees. Above all, trees. They're magnificent and fill you up with wonder.

There again, get out of the house by doing something you've always wanted to. You could join a political party and sample a local political meeting. If archery is something you've always wanted to do, don't hesitate. Get the gear and go along to the local club. If you've always had a yen to paint or sculpt, enrol at a local evening class.

You might yearn to go on an exotic cruise. Book one now and imagine yourself making on-board friendships with new and likeminded people. Or consider a cruise down the Nile or around the Greek Islands where you can see new sights, soak up new cultures, and learn at the same time. Some such tours can be cheaper than you realise – and if you have the money to treat yourself, do it!

M

Make-Up

I'M NOT A FAN OF a five-point plan on how to take care of your skin often recommended at beauty counters and online. My skin care routine is much simpler than that and has been refined over many years. Really, I have only two steps, cleansing and moisturising.

I feel I must nail my colours to the mast and say, I'm a fan of make-up and have been since the age of 15 when I first applied a pale pink lipstick. It wasn't pale enough for my dad, however. He was horrified and took me to the kitchen sink, placed my head under the tap and washed off the lipstick with carbolic soap. This silliness didn't put me off. I love the idea that my face is a blank canvas which I could paint and shape with foundation, blushers, and highlighters.

From the beginning I loved eye make-up, believing the eyes are the windows of the soul and should be emphasised in every face. It wasn't just the dressing up aspect of make-up that thrilled me. I found the world of cosmetics an exciting Aladdin's cave. Being a good student, I studied make-up a lot. I followed articles in women's magazines, I avidly devoured information on new trends, I studied how models made up their eyes and tried out new ideas endlessly. I studied so hard I could have been a PhD student in make-up. I'm ready to admit that in those early days I felt myself not quite up to the mark with my other girlfriends who were confident and outgoing and make-up made me feel "more equal" and more confident. More than that, make-up made me feel I could compete.

When much later I became a dermatologist, I realised that make-up was one of the best ways to keep your skin moisturised, plump and wrinkle-free. It retains moisture in the skin. In fact, it's one the most efficient moisturisers and its effect lasts as long as your make-up is on your skin. One of the practices that grew out of this knowledge was that I didn't routinely take my make-up off at the end of the day. Leaving it on could keep my skin moisturised for as long as I left the make-up on. I know, I know, I know. My approach to make-up isn't everybody's cup of tea. When I tell people that I haven't washed my face since the age of 15, they're horrified but the water that comes out of most of our taps is, paradoxically, dehydrating. It dries out the skin because it contains salts which draw moisture out of the skin. Just think of the wrinkles in your fingertips if you stay in the bath too long.

Soap is another no-no. In addition to drying out the skin it de-fats the skin and removes the protective, oily mantle, which covers all our skin and which is slightly acidic. The skin enjoys being slightly acidic and anything on the alkaline side is detrimental to the health of the skin.

As I approach my 90s I think make-up is still important. Partly because it does my skin good and partly because I still want to make the best of myself. To my mind that's not frivolous, it's not arrogant, it's not a waste of time and it's not vain. I'm just paying a little attention to presentation. All through our lives we concentrate on presentation, whether it's a piece of work for your boss or if it's polishing the apples for your child to put on the school nature table in the autumn. I'm aware that many women will disagree not only with my approach to make-up but also the importance I give it. That's fine. The information here is for anyone who feels they could benefit from it and is comfortable with giving it a go.

Rest assured, putting on make-up needn't be time consuming. From start to finish, my routine takes 40 minutes so not a big investment. I still look forward to my make-up sessions with the latest products that make use of clever science. It still remains fun and I still like experimenting with new cosmetics. I still look at models to see how they're making up their eyes.

By and large I don't use expensive cosmetics. I refuse to pay for costly advertising campaigns and expensive packaging. All I'm interested in are the ingredients and I remain sceptical about the claims made for expensive products, however persuasive the selling line sounds. There's always a cheaper alternative, and it's probably as equally effective as the expensive one.

The cleansing products I use are at the cheap end of the Boots cosmetic aisle. First, a two-phase liquid cleanser on a cotton wool pad to remove my make-up, I use Nivea, followed by a splash of micellar water (Garnier). Then I hydrate. I've used many different moisturisers over the years but I'm stuck on the comparatively new serums. There are a lot of expensive ones around but you can get an excellent one cheaply from Boots. Being a sceptic I never expect products to fulfil the promises they make, but serums do. Almost all contain hyaluronic acid which is a potent moisturiser, dragging moisture into the skin and keeping it there. It plumps up collagen and really does smooth out wrinkles. If you're lucky, this effect can last up to 18 hours. The plumping action can result in a mild peel which gets rid of dead skin cells and leaves a smooth sparkling skin surface to apply your make-up.

Learning to use cosmetics with any degree of success takes time and effort and I've put in my 10,000 hours practising to achieve the look I want. Over the years I've been fortunate enough to pick up good tips from TV make-up experts. Years ago I learned one technique from a make-up guy in New York where I was going to be interviewed on the midday television news. He wasn't very complimentary.

"Your face is very round so we have to try to slim it down with blusher. So I'll sweep the blusher right up to the outer corner of your eye and give you cheekbones to make your face look longer."

I liked the result and incorporated the technique into my make-up routine. I've used it ever since and still do to this day.

I love the paraphernalia of make-up and have found using brushes gives the best results. I use brushes for everything as they give much better coverage than fingertips and are more accurate.

Here's my equipment:

- The brushes I use to smooth in foundation are very soft, long-handled and blunt-tipped to get into all the crevices. You may opt for some lip brushes which are the most accurate tool for applying lip colour.
- Contour brushes to apply powder, blushes and shaders.
- Eye shadow brushes or sponge-tipped applicators for powdered shadow. You'll need one for each of the different colours you use.
- An eyebrow brush to train eyebrows and brush off excess powder.
- Small sponges to apply liquid make-up. Mac does excellent ones.
- Clean powder puffs for applying loose and compressed face powder. Personally I've grown out of loose powder and now I only use pressed or "blot" powder. There are good ones by Mac and Clinique.
- Q-tips for fine blending, removing excess and tidying up lines and mistakes.
- I also have on hand eyebrow tweezers, cosmetic pencil sharpeners plus an array of eyeliner pencils. I like the soft ones done by Laura Mercier and never black – brown and grey.
- Liquid eyeliners in brown and grey, never black.

I learned from a make-up artist to do my eye make-up first before doing anything else. It makes sense because when applying powder eye shadow it's hard to avoid little specks falling onto your cheeks which are difficult to remove and may spoil your make-up. So my make-up starts off with my eyes. My routine is one that I've refined over many years. It's extremely simple. I apply a stick eyeshadow over the whole of my upper eyelid and blend it a little into the eye socket. I also blend it underneath the eye. When the blending is complete I "set it" by using a little pressed powder on a small soft brush. I can't overemphasise the importance of "setting" the make-up. Once set it won't budge and needs no touching up.

The next step is to apply foundation. My favourite is CC cream, the CC standing for complexion correcting which I need now, as my skin is old and has many imperfections and broken veins. I use a colour which is one shade lighter than my natural skin colour. This is because as we grow older our skin becomes sallow and a lighter shade enlivens it.

The foundation provides a base for the rest of my make-up and helps protect my skin. I then apply blot powder from Mac to set the foundation. I brush on powder until my skin doesn't feel tacky. Next comes blusher to emphasise the cheekbones and put a little colour on the apple of my cheeks.

Then comes eyebrow make-up and I like Benefit products. I've never plucked my eyebrows because I don't like the plucked look, nor do I like the look of the eyebrows painted on the face. I put the finishing touches to my eyes with a waterline pencil and mascara. It's a long time since I used black eyeliner in the waterline or mascara because I find it ages the face. The effect is too harsh, so I only use brown or grey. The final touch is my lips and I take particular care of them because as we get older lines form around our lips and lipstick can easily seep into these lines which is something I try to avoid. I do this by using a great product from Mac which is called Lip Primer. It's a stick of wax which you put around the outline of your mouth so your lipstick doesn't bleed. I apply it and leave it for 10 minutes to set then I know I can apply either a lip outliner pencil or lipstick on its own and it will still be intact after several hours.

How long should you keep your make-up for?

Yes, we're all guilty of using expired make-up and it's definitely not good for the skin. Here are a few products and how often you should change them.

Liquid foundation – use it for a year but discard it earlier if a clear liquid forms on top or its texture changes.
Eye pencil – this one is a keeper as long as you clean the tip after every use or sharpen it to take off the top layer. If you're a liquid eyeliner fan, change it every six months.
Mascara – it should be changed every six months or sooner if it starts to smell, to avoid eye infection.
Lipstick – they're usually good for about a year but if it smells or it's difficult to apply, it's time for a new one.

Masturbation, Vibrators & Orgasms

THIS SECTION IS REALLY AN overview of orgasms, but I've focussed it on masturbation and vibrators because they are the sure-fire way to bring yourself to orgasm.

Now's the time to embrace vibrators! Yes, now that you're getting on there's little room for prudishness and you've earned the right to be adventurous, even if you're not curious. The daughter of a friend told me that her mother (my friend, a widow of a similar age to me) in response to the question, "What would you like for your birthday, Mum?" replied with, "A vibrator". I know my friend to be a curious, adventurous, life-loving woman. She clearly didn't want to miss out on trying a vibrator before it was too late, and nor should you.

In my earlier pregnancy books and my sex book I encouraged women to masturbate (men need no encouragement, they do it all the time, from a young age). But I've met women who'd had several children and never had an orgasm. I remember speaking to a 78-year-old New Yorker who'd never had an orgasm in all her married life but recently had started orgasming with a new boyfriend, a toy boy. Well, you needn't start looking for a toy boy, just buy a vibrator. Orgasms are guaranteed.

We're all of us made differently "down there" and we have our own particular sweet spots (not the so-called G spot), on and around the clitoris. If you aren't familiar with your anatomy stop reading now, look it up on the internet immediately. Better still, get a mirror and take a look at yours.

Most clitorises find masturbation and vibrators, particularly vibrators, irresistible. So if you didn't start masturbating when you were 10, 11, 12 and don't know what an orgasm is like, start masturbating now and using a vibrator. No one can know our anatomy, our trigger points and pleasure spots like we can ourselves. So it's up to you to find out and then share your knowledge with a loving partner if you are in a relationship. If you are single then vibrators and masturbation are the way to enjoy orgasms alone.

We all have the right to orgasms, we're sexual animals and it's up to you not to miss out on them. This is where vibrators come in. Orgasms can be both elusive and fleeting. Vibrators allow you to overcome both things. A vibrator can guarantee an orgasm every time and prolong an orgasm that's often over too quickly. Best of all, you're in control.

I remember writing in one of my pregnancy books that you should continue to have sex right through pregnancy because with all those hormones, reproductive and sexual, flying around you'll have the most intense orgasms you've ever had. The same, I've discovered, can happen as we get older using a vibrator. And there's the bonus that orgasms need not be elusive but ever ready in our older years.

I've pondered this phenomenon and I can tell you why I think this is. If you've had a rich sex life through most of your life the nerve pathways from your vagina and clitoris to your brain and nervous system that culminate in orgasm are well-worn and familiar. The sexual sensations can whizz with ever-increasing ease and speed towards orgasm as you go through your 60s, 70s, 80s, and yes, 90s. So if you want, you can have the most intense orgasms of your life as you get older, alone or with a partner. Who would miss out on that? And this rich sexual future is just waiting there for anyone who would like to live it. I realise you have to be more open about your sexuality than perhaps you've ever been and that may not be easy for you. Have you thought that one of the best things awaiting you in your older years is being a free sexual spirit? What an unexpected joy and it's available to all of us if we're brave enough. The good news is if you thought that getting older meant a gradual withdrawal into a sexless life you'd be wrong. Your sex life can be richer than ever. Welcome it!

This empowering, enriching discovery can free you from worry about sex, and freedom from performance anxiety. You may not have orgasms every time, but so what? It's no big deal, now you know how to orgasm. Embracing masturbation, vibrators and orgasming at will frees you from embarrassment about erection problems, erectile dysfunction, new relationships, broaching sex with a new partner. Accepting yourself as a sexual being is one key to being confident and outgoing, making friends, joining clubs, taking up new hobbies, travelling, being a fun grandparent, learning a new skill, studying a new language, improved self-worth and loving yourself.

Maybe that's the person you've always wanted to be.

Microbiome

THE WORD MICROBIOME IS COMPARATIVELY new. Even before there was the word, I recognised there were several places in the body which, in retrospect, could be described as having a "microbiome". The vagina, for instance, is populated by a community of bacteria, fungi (candida) and viruses that live in harmony together without causing any disease; in fact they keep the vagina healthy. Similarly, we knew about the trillions of bacteria living in the gut that are an essential part of our immune system and again, live happily together promoting health. We also know any disturbance of these flourishing communities of microbes can end up with disease. So, for instance, the use of vaginal deodorants will disturb the vaginal microbiome causing vaginosis, unwanted growth of bacteria with soreness, itchiness, and discharge.

Similarly, antibiotics will upset the finely tuned balance of microbes in the gut, allowing certain bacteria to overgrow and cause symptoms like diarrhoea. When the microbiome of the gut is disturbed by antibiotics, one of the clearest signs is thrush, an overgrowth of the fungus, candida. This happens because the bacterial community in the gut is partly destroyed, allowing candida to overgrow. In fact, other organs have "microbiomes" like the mouth and the external ear, and disruption of them can cause symptoms.

We've found the gut microbiome performs functions way beyond anything we imagined when it was first described. We know, for instance, that a certain type of microbiome predisposes to putting on weight and this can be counteracted with a "faecal implant" from somebody whose microbiome doesn't predispose to weight gain.

Looking after your gut microbiome

- Never take antibiotics unless your GP prescribes them and then take them as instructed and finish the course.
- **Probiotics** – good bacteria – may be helpful in some cases, such as preventing diarrhoea and with some symptoms of irritable bowel syndrome (IBS) but there's little evidence to support many other health claims made about them.
- Fibre is a **prebiotic** – it feeds good bacteria – so incorporate more fibre in your diet in the form of fruits, vegetables, and whole grains and cut down on processed, fatty and sugary foods.

Several drinks can support gut health by giving you beneficial bacteria. These are probiotics drinks like kefir, kombucha, herbal teas like peppermint and ginger, and water – they are all good choices. Kefir is a fermented milk rich in probiotics, so can help improve gut health. Kombucha is another fermented drink made by fermenting sweetened tea with probiotic bacteria. Buttermilk contains probiotics and lactic acid which improve gut health and digestion. And then there are the commercial probiotic drinks. Actimel is known to be beneficial and that's the one I drink, not every day, just when I remember. The microbiome loves fermenting foods and so thrives on kimchi and sauerkraut.

You can also support your gut by eating and drinking prebiotic foods which provide fibre for the good bacteria in your gut to live on and thrive. All fruit and vegetables are prebiotics because of the fibre they contain, especially green bananas and berries, vegetables like onion, garlic, leeks, artichokes, asparagus and other root vegetables are also full of fibre. Legumes like chickpeas, lentils and beans are good additions to your diet, as are wholegrains like oats, rye, barley and wheat, plus nuts such as pistachios, cashews, almonds and seeds.

Here are a few more prebiotic foods: Jerusalem artichokes, chicory root, dandelion greens, onions, leeks, asparagus, bananas, barley, oats, apples, flax seeds, wheat bran, seaweed, avocado. Since the fibre content of these foods may be altered by cooking, try to eat them raw to gain the full health benefits. It's worth taking time to find the best prebiotic foods for yourself and your gut.

For optimal health and to keep your microbiome healthy, eat a variety of foods, at least 30 different foods each week. Choose wholefoods, if possible, fresh and uncooked. Remember staying hydrated is important for your digestion and so is regular exercise which can affect your microbiome for the good.

Your microbiome impacts on all aspects of your health. It not only influences digestion but it affects immune function and brain function. The staggering fact is that 70% of our immune system is in the microbiome in our gut.

The contribution of the microbiome to our health is critical – it helps protect the body from harmful bacteria by releasing its own antibiotics and strengthening the body's defences against infection. It reduces the risk of autoimmune disease and it interacts with the brain via the gut-brain axis by producing neurotransmitters such as serotonin that can affect brain function and mood. An imbalance in the microbiome has been linked to various mental health conditions, including anxiety, depression, even neurological disorders.

It plays an important role in regulating blood sugar levels and insulin sensitivity, potentially lowering the risk for type 2 diabetes.

It also affects the way we use calories, possibly contributing to obesity if its function is weakened. The gut microbiome has also been linked to various other health conditions, including heart disease, inflammatory bowel disease, and even certain types of cancer. The following have been linked to gut bacteria imbalance: autoimmune problems such as thyroid issues, rheumatoid arthritis and type 1 diabetes. Digestive issues such as irritable bowel syndrome, constipation, diarrhoea and heartburn and bloating are other possibilities. Signs of an unhealthy gut microbiome are bloating and gas, and general symptoms like fatigue, skin problems and mood changes.

Mindfulness

PUT SIMPLY, MINDFULNESS MEANS LIVING in the moment and accepting what you see at face value without making any judgments. I think this acceptance is an important part of mindfulness because your mind goes into neutral and that's restful and nourishing. It's a relief for your brain. By focusing on what you're seeing you become aware of what you're feeling, letting your thoughts roam free without curbing them and you become aware of any physical sensations that unfold without wanting to analyse or control them.

Mindfulness is seen as a kind of meditation where you might incorporate special breathing, imagery and visualisation, yoga to help you relax your body and mind and help to make it easier to deal with stress.

I'm a great believer in meditation and mindfulness. I find myself practising mindfulness whenever I leave the house, instinctively pausing to look at what surrounds me and also to listen to the sounds around me. The benefits of meditation are well-researched and there's good evidence that it may help relieve stress, anxiety, pain, depression, insomnia, and high blood pressure[32].

The cardinal elements of mindfulness are to pay attention to what your senses are relaying to you, and not just visual, but sound, smell, taste and touch. So a good example would be to focus on what you're eating, roll the taste around your mouth and connect with the feeling and the sensations that it brings to you. Living in the moment gives you an open and spontaneous approach to everything you see and do. And spontaneity brings such joy. I remember once my husband was punting me along a quiet English river and we came across someone who was fishing. As I come from a fishing family, I recognised his rod, which was unusual. It was a particular type of pole used for roach fishing. I'd never seen one before and as we glided past, I said to the fisherman, "Are the roach biting today?". For a few moments, my husband stopped punting and said, "Miri, where does your spontaneity come from?". The only answer I had for him was I notice what's going on around me and if something is particularly interesting, I comment.

The other aspect of mindfulness is something which all of us find quite difficult, accepting ourselves as we are. To my mind, by the time we've reached our 60s, we've earned the right to be who we are. That acceptance can bring great contentment.

I'm an inveterate "breather" by which I mean I believe in the calming effect of concentrating on your breathing. You'll feel calmer still if you cut your breathing rate in half and concentrate on each breath. I close my eyes, halve my breathing rate and then breathe in for a count of five, hold my breath for a count of five and breathe out for the same length. As I do it, I can feel my pulse rate slackening and my blood pressure coming down.

---

[32] https://www.nccih.nih.gov/health/meditation-and-mindfulness-effectiveness-and-safety

Sex, Drugs & Walking Sticks

Money Worries

THERE ARE PRECIOUS FEW PEOPLE over 60 who have no money worries at all. People who have carefully planned for their life after retirement by taking out substantial life insurance that will cover their cost of living and allows some spare for luxuries, are small in number. Generally, the financial outlook for the over 60s is perilous. The stats say it all and there are plenty of them. Over 90% of people in this age group are worried about the cost of living and 25% in the 50+ age group are severely affected by money worries. Research shows poor health is intimately related to financial hardship. There are very strong links between "wealth and health"[33].

As we get older it's not uncommon to be forced to cut back and make sacrifices at the expense of physical and mental health. People are delaying retirement or going back to work, they're socialising less and travelling less because the costs are no longer affordable. Subsequent isolation from friends and family results in loneliness. Because of reduced disposable income, many people are having to cut back on the support they get with cleaning, gardening, household chores and hygiene. They eat less and spend less.

One in five 50+ people are skipping meals and using savings to pay bills. Loss of disposable income is the most common financial worry and 80% in the 65+ age group believe the state pension isn't enough to cover costs. Furthermore, one in five 60-64-year-olds are living in deep poverty[34]. While poverty in later life has always

---

33   https://www.ageuk.org.uk/discover/2024/march/the-link-between-wealth-and-health/

34   https://www.independentage.org/news-media/press-releases/too-little-too-late-state-pension-and-social-security-safety-net-failing

existed, it's the highest it's been since 2007. In people nearing retirement, two-thirds aren't confident that retirement income would cover their rent. For some, retirement isn't even an option. Some older people are missing out on financial support, such as the Pension Credit, which rounds up income to a minimum level, housing benefit, attendance allowance, and carers allowance. Many benefits may exist, but to an older person access to them may be so complicated that they find it impossible to take advantage of them. Frankly, to find one's way through the tortuous route of accessing state benefits I think you should speak to a benefit advisor who will be available from your local council and take a young family member with you. In this way you'll make sure that you're not missing out on any benefits that you qualify for.

It's very clear that having sufficient income to live adequately in old age requires planning and to plan early on, way before retirement is on the horizon. So conversations with a partner to discuss financial options that could provide income in later years are a necessity. Parents should probably have discussions with the family, with their children so that a secure financial future can be mapped out for them. If you're still in work, of course, your pension has to be negotiated with your employer, though there are legal requirements of your employer in this situation.

The people who are in the fortunate position of having planned for their retirement or who have assets that will fund their retirement are relatively small in number. A woman who has been widowed may have to wait a very long time for the completion of probation on her husband's will before she receives any financial support from it. This can leave her without any income at all for two or three years, unless she takes out loans or is helped by the rest of the family.

Retirees with enough money to support their way of life would be wise to budget carefully and make sure that a surviving partner has adequate funds to live on their own. Grandparents who wish to contribute to the cost of education of their grandchildren will have to plan carefully and budget for those expenses.

The impact of the cost of living crisis on coping financially during retirement isn't all bad news. According to a 2024 report from the FCA (Financial Conduct Authority)[35], the UK's retired population appears to be coping better with the cost of living crisis than their younger counterparts. A survey of 3,450 people found more than two-fifths (41%) of those over 75, and around a third (34%) of people aged 65-74, were financially managing themselves very well.

They're doing better than 19-34-year-olds where more than a third (35%) admitted not coping financially during the cost of living crisis, with just 6% believing they're managing very well.

How to make your pension go further

Downsize

The single biggest saving you can make is downsizing your property. If it's just you and your partner in the family home you might want to think about moving into a smaller house where your bills and maintenance will be much less and you'll have cash to put into your retirement savings. Sometimes people may feel anxious about leaving a family home where they feel settled but it could be a good opportunity to move to a property which will be more suitable in the longer term and with good public transport links.

Track your spending

Create a spreadsheet (or get help to create one) with all your outgoings and track it every month to make sure you're not overspending. People tend to think they spend less than they actually

---

[35] https://www.fca.org.uk/publication/financial-lives/financial-lives-cost-of-living-jan-2024-recontact-survey-findings.pdf

do so keeping an eye on your outgoings will show you where your money is being spent and where you can save some cash.

Use public transport

Having a car in retirement could cost a lot so, if you're able, consider using public transport instead. You can apply for a Senior Railcard which will give you a third off on train ticket purchases. If you live in London you can apply for a Freedom Pass to use public transport for free any time Monday to Friday, except between 04:30-09:00, and on weekends and bank holidays.

Have a part-time job

Getting a job, even if only for a few hours a week, would supplement your pension and lessen your money worries. A part-time job would give framework to your day – going to work, meeting colleagues plus keeping your brain agile.

Moving home

Before making any big decisions, sit down and think about the implications of your move, such as do you want to move into a flat, bungalow, sheltered accommodation or a care home. Involve your whole family in the decision making and take steps to stay in contact with family and old friends.

N

Norovirus

THIS IS THE "WINTER VOMITING bug" which quite often affects close groups of children in schools and nurseries. It's contagious and can rip through a school. It's a stomach bug that causes vomiting and diarrhoea and can be very unpleasant both in children and adults. I'm including it here because anything that causes vomiting or diarrhoea in an older person may cause dehydration rapidly with dizziness, headache and unsteadiness, and has to be treated quickly. Dehydration has serious consequences, lowering your blood pressure as it does, giving your heart more work to do even possibly depriving your brain of oxygen.

If you've had contact with a child or someone who has the norovirus your symptoms will probably appear between 12 and 48 hours after your exposure. Symptoms such as feeling sick, nausea and vomiting can strike you out of the blue. You may also have watery diarrhoea, stomach cramps and possibly a mild fever.

Norovirus causes symptoms which are similar to flu with aching joints and limbs, headaches and general tiredness. Some people may only have mild symptoms like nausea and get better quite quickly. Even though the infection is usually over in one to three days some people may be contagious for longer, possibly up to two weeks after their recovery because while the symptoms have abated, the virus can still be shed in stools. Norovirus is so contagious that if one person in your family gets it, other members of your family may get it too.

There's no specific antiviral treatment for norovirus, so treatment is focused on relieving your symptoms. It's essential to keep hydrated by drinking a lot of fluids such as water or clear soup. If you have diarrhoea as well drink oral rehydration solutions so that you don't run short of important electrolytes like sodium and potassium. Help your body to recover by resting. Don't glug down a glass of water, instead take small, frequent sips and ease back into eating with very plain food such as some tea with dry toast, bland and easy to digest foods such as crackers, soup, oats, noodles, bananas and rice can be introduced slowly when you feel like it.

The norovirus has the ability to persist on hard and soft surfaces so it's important to disinfect surfaces and wash bedding frequently. On hard surfaces the virus may persist for two weeks. Be meticulous about hand hygiene when you use a public restroom. The average hand sanitiser is ineffective against the norovirus as are alcohol-based sanitisers but chlorine-based sanitisers are effective. Generally, Imodium isn't recommended for relieving diarrhoea in norovirus infection and antibiotics don't help.

Lucozade isn't recommended as a rehydration drink for norovirus as it contains too much sugar. Rehydration solutions like Dioralyte or Pedialyte are much superior. Good old porridge is a good choice to eat after vomiting as it's bland, starchy and easy on the stomach. When you make it, use extra water so that it's thinner and will keep you hydrated.

The norovirus with diarrhoea doesn't wipe out your microbiome completely and it will recover over time. Norovirus isn't primarily transmitted in droplets in the air like Covid and flu, it's usually passed on by direct contact with someone who has the infection. Once you get norovirus, all you can do is to let the virus run its course and you should try to protect the other people around you from catching it by staying at home. In terms of settling your stomach, the best foods are boiled potatoes, rice, and noodles. Repopulate your gut microbiome afterwards with kefir, kombucha and Actimel.

O

Optimism

IT MAY BE HARD TO believe, but your attitude to life helps you stay healthy and live longer so it's worth trying to stay positive if you can. As we get older, that's not always easy to do and we need self-affirming thoughts (see next page) to stay on top of things but having an optimistic frame of mind can give you real resilience as you get older. I'm sure you can think of people who always look on the bright side, think every cloud has a silver lining, and believe better times will come tomorrow. This kind of optimism is a great healer. There's quite a lot of research showing that people who can stay positive have not only fewer illnesses but also recover more quickly when they are ill[36].

One of the great attributes of optimism is that it helps you feel you can take charge of your life and your health. You can be proactive when you grow old and not dwindle into old age. If you look at the lifestyle of optimists, you find they're really looking after themselves "because they're worth it". They eat well, exercise enough, don't smoke, and drink only in moderation. Not surprisingly they rarely get depressed. Not only do they tend to live longer, but they seem to be comfortable with getting older. Thinking positively and

---

36 https://newsinhealth.nih.gov/2015/08/positive-emotions-your-health#:~:text=Research%20has%20found%20a%20link,sugar%20levels%2C%20and%20longer%20life

making the most of your inner resources will help to keep your optimistic nature and so will these positive thoughts, as they apply to you. Thoughts such as these…

- My life belongs to me and I enjoy it.
- I get through my work efficiently and competently.
- I'm learning to handle stress little by little.
- I eat healthy, nourishing food most of the time.
- I exercise enough to keep my body in good condition.
- I'm generally calm and relaxed.
- I have the freedom and confidence to be adventurous.
- I give time to myself every day and look after myself.
- I can be happy and optimistic at this time of my life.
- My friends and family are closer than ever.

Try not to think any of these statements as impossible. They aren't. Repeat them every day like a mantra and you'll come to believe them. Towards this end write them out and pin them to the fridge door. Every time you open it say a couple of them to yourself.

More people than you might think have an optimistic view of their life, and the future, when they reach their 70s and 80s. A study of 10,000 people aged between 15-90 carried out over four consecutive years by gerontologist Professor Ian Stuart-Hamilton and an expert on the scientific study of ageing, to understand the psychological aspects of ageing, concluded that the old chestnut about older people being devoid of fun is not true.

And in support of this, he says more and more septuagenarians are enjoying life and retiring late, sometimes not until they're over 70. (If writing this book qualifies as work, neither have I.) Even when these people, having worked all their lives, retire, they go on to have full social lives. Even more reassuring is research showing the overall satisfaction with life of people in their 90s is greater than people half their age. The truth is that contentment with most aspects of life improves with age along with a greater sense of well-being. Could this be because older people know how to enjoy down time? Turns out when you're 35 you're least likely to be happy with the amount of leisure time you have, whereas the over 70s are the most satisfied.

The power of optimism

Why am I banging on about optimism? While there's no single elixir of life there's lots of research to show that optimists live longer than pessimists sometimes becoming "super agers"[37]. People who can grasp the positives from even dire events will enjoy more years of life.

When I saw the film *Youth*, with the wonderful Michael Caine, I was struck by the simple, but profound message – resilience and optimism are crucial ingredients of long life, fulfilment and happiness.

In fact if I had to choose one factor that would help give me a long, healthy life it would be optimism. It confers real resilience as you get older and it's a great healer. Optimists take charge of their health and refuse to slide into old age. As a rule they take better care of themselves. They exercise regularly, sleep better, but don't drink or smoke too much, and are generally free from depression. They age more gradually and live longer. Pessimism, on the other hand, is not good for you. Pessimists have high levels of T-suppressor cells which weakens the immune system. Negativity and hopelessness are accompanied by a greater risk of heart disease.

Contentment rises as we get older with a peak at 70 and people up to the age of 90 still register a higher score of satisfaction with life than people half their age. Why? Well, there's time for

---

37   https://www.pnas.org/doi/10.1073/pnas.1900712116

sightseeing, time for travelling, for taking skiing holidays, for spending weeks on trekking in the Himalayas, for the trip to the Antarctic you've always longed for or for the simple pleasures of a walk in the countryside or pottering in the garden. People who've experienced life appreciate what it has to offer and are grateful for what they can still do. Seventy-year-olds are still enthusiastic about life. This may be because older people know how to enjoy their leisure time.

What's surprising, however, is how strong the effect is. Among 160,000 participants in the Woman's Health Initiative, optimism was associated with a 5% increase in life span, adding an average of four years of life[38]. That's comparable to the benefits of exercise!

There are some things you can do to be more optimistic. For instance, do more of what excites you and motivates you. Make a bucket list of things you "must" do in the rest of your life and tick them off. Read about people who've accomplished things in the second half of their lives. Find yourself a role model and imitate them. Concentrate on your strengths and forget your weaknesses.

How to be an optimist and live longer

I've written many times that optimists live longer than pessimists. But what if you're not a natural optimist? Can you learn optimism?

Well, you can if you believe in the work of Dr Barbara Fredrickson, psychologist at the University of North Carolina who's done great work on how to promote positive emotions. I particularly like her theory that accumulating "micro-moments of positivity," can lead to well-being. She believes that collecting positive emotions from everyday activities can decide who lives a long life and who doesn't. Her research shows[39] the accumulation of brief moments

---

38 https://hsph.harvard.edu/news/optimism-longevity-women/
39 https://pmc.ncbi.nlm.nih.gov/articles/PMC3126102/

of positive feelings can protect us against stress and depression, keeping us physically and mentally healthy. Brief moments like enjoying a sunset, savouring a nice cup of tea, laughing at a joke and going for a walk in the park.

When we have negative feelings a region of the brain called the amygdala is activated and we become fearful and anxious. Researchers have shown a person can learn to be more positive by practising certain skills that foster positivity and generate new brain cells and pathways. So it is possible to train the circuitry in the brain to be more positive.

So much so that Dr Fredrickson's six weeks of training in compassion meditation leads to more friendly behaviour towards others and better heart rate control. In turn, this results in better control of blood glucose, less inflammation and faster recovery from a heart attack. In fact as little as two weeks' training in compassion and kindness meditation promotes brain changes linked to being friendly and generous.

The researchers believe: "…positive emotions can help us become healthier, more social, more resilient versions of ourselves". And Dr Fredrickson believes if two people can share these positive moments it's even better for our health and happiness.

Osteoporosis

ALL THE BONES IN OUR bodies are affected by age. One in five post-menopausal women will have some osteoporosis. This is a gradual thinning and softening of the bones caused by loss of calcium and protein, pursuant on the cut-off of the female hormones, oestrogen and progesterone, at the menopause.

The word osteoporosis means "bone that has many holes", consequently it's brittle and vulnerable to fractures. That's because with age our bone repairing system weakens. Let me explain. When we're young, worn out bone gets broken down by cells called osteoclasts and repaired by cells called osteoblasts. This fine balance of removing and building bone keeps our skeleton strong and solid. But for about 15 years after the menopause, bone is removed faster than it's replaced causing osteoporosis, leaving it vulnerable to fracture. Without the boost of HRT a woman will lose 30% of her bone mass within three years of her periods stopping.

Without regular weight-bearing exercise, osteoporosis will get worse with age, making bones more likely to break, particularly the wrists, hips and spine, sometimes leading to curvature of the spine. Osteoporosis is responsible for 500,000 fractures each year, commonly to the hip, wrist and spine[40].

Are women especially at risk?

Osteoporosis starts as early as 50 when oestrogen levels begin to fall. Without oestrogen bones get brittle and snap. That's painful, but worse, it can be fatal – one in four women who go into hospital with a hip fracture due to osteoporosis never come out – they die there. Osteoporosis isn't an exclusively female problem – men suffer from it too.

Prevention is paramount

In 2022, it was estimated that the cost of treating a fractured hip was £11,905[41]. Add to that the cost of care and it's clear we're dealing with a disease which not only causes terrible pain and is potentially life threatening but it's also a huge challenge for our

---

40   https://www.nhsinform.scot/illnesses-and-conditions/muscle-bone-and-joints/conditions-that-can-affect-multiple-parts-of-the-body/osteoporosis/
41   https://research-information.bris.ac.uk/en/publications/up-to-date-costs-of-hip-fracture-care-in-england-and-wales-identi

NHS. Far better to prevent osteoporosis from developing or to halt its progress with a good diet, daily exercise, vitamin D and calcium before it gets too bad.

If you succeed...
- You'll avoid fractured hips and hip replacement.
- Your bones won't break if you fall.
- You'll avoid bone and joint pain.
- You won't get a collapsed spine and a Dowager's Hump.

Watch out for grey hair before your 40s

Premature grey hair could be a sign of bone thinning. Grey hair before the age of 40 is indicative of thin bones. So premature grey hair could be an invaluable risk marker for osteoporosis. If your hair goes grey before you're 40 check your bone health with your doctor.

How to keep your bones young

The mainstays of healthy bones are weight-bearing exercise like walking and a diet rich in calcium, vitamin D in supplement form, 10mcg a day from October-April.

Diet
- Increase your calcium intake by eating calcium-rich foods, like dairy products and canned fish with bones, such as sardines. Taking vitamin D during the dark winter months will maximise calcium absorption.
- Choose low-fat milk and dairy products containing calcium.
- The body finds it difficult to absorb calcium without vitamin D. Natural vitamin D is in oily fish such as sardines, herring and mackerel, then there's fortified cereals, bread and margarine. Cod liver oil capsules are also a good source.

Exercise

To me the evidence in favour of exercise is irresistible. People who take exercise twice a week have denser bones than those who exercise only once a week, who, in turn, have denser bones than those who don't take exercise at all. There's a significant improvement in bone strength for women who exercise for half an hour three times a week.

The Osteoporosis Society suggests the following exercises which you might like to try.

The first is the shoulder squeeze: While sitting on the edge of a chair pull your arms upwards, outwards and back, so that you squeeze your shoulder blades together. Stay like that for three to five seconds and do them again eight to 10 times.

The second one is a yoga pose called the "cat/cow". Get down on the floor in a table top position. While breathing out, lower your stomach towards the floor and lift your bum up. Hold this position for five seconds. On your second exhale pull your stomach in and arch your back up curling your head and chin down as far as you can. Stay like that for five seconds and repeat eight to 10 times.

How to lower your chances of brittle bones

- Don't let yourself get too thin.
- Eat foods containing calcium and vitamin D.
- Take plenty of weight bearing exercise e.g. walking.
- Don't smoke.
- Keep alcohol consumption low.
- Eat dark green leafy vegetables.
- Don't eat much red meat.
- Eat foods containing magnesium like almonds, peanuts, banana, spinach, low-fat dairy.
- Keep salt intake low.

Drugs for osteoporosis

The most commonly used drugs for osteoporosis are bisphosphonates which slow down bone breakdown. Other commonly used drugs are denosumab, raloxifene, and calcitonin which have different mechanisms of action to strengthen bones and maintain bone density. I sustained two fractures of my lower spine because of the jolt to my body when I jumped off a high wall. Immediately afterwards I felt nothing. But the next morning I couldn't walk at all and the pain was agonising. An MRI scan showed two cracks in my sacrum. Recovery was very slow and I wasn't able to walk normally for six weeks. I'm on denosumab (Prolia) which is a monoclonal antibody, a biological drug which stops bone breakdown and thereby strengthens bones. Others such as alendronic acid and Risedronate may be used if you can't take the others. Alendronic acid (Fosamax) is most often prescribed to prevent spine fracture by strengthening bones. The latest drugs for osteoporosis are Abaloparatide and Romosozumab (an injection), another monoclonal antibody for people with a high risk of bone fracture and those who don't respond to other treatments.

P

Pain & Pain Management

PAIN THAT LASTS MORE THAN a few days is debilitating and exhausting. As we get older and our tissues start to wear out, pain of some sort may become a daily occurrence, making life difficult. Pain may be naturally limited, for instance, some kinds of back pain which resolve themselves within six weeks or so. On the other hand, when back pain becomes chronic (persistent) it's much more difficult to treat and needs careful management. We'll be jolly lucky if at some point in our older age we don't have to cope with chronic pain which needs managing as well as treating.

Treatment is part of management, but management is more comprehensive than just treatment. A mainstay of acute treatment is painkillers such as paracetamol and NSAIDs (non-steroidal anti-inflammatory drugs) both of which, used properly, can bring relief. The simplest treatment, paracetamol, is powerful and efficient if used precisely – taking a gram (two tablets) every four hours. There's a general understanding between doctors and patients that even for severe pain, opioids, narcotics, should be avoided at all costs because they're addictive.

For chronic pain which lasts months, even years, your doctor might refer you to a specialised pain clinic where a number of specialists with an interest in pain management work together to find solutions for you and draw up a management plan.

A pain management plan is wide-ranging and may stretch into many aspects of your daily life. For instance, the basis of all pain management is living a healthy lifestyle, watching weight, being as physically active as is possible, eating a healthy diet, avoiding pain triggers, and paying attention to posture at all times. Chronic pain is helped by a lot more than painkillers. There's plenty of research showing keeping a healthy weight, exercising regularly, by that I mean a daily walk, avoiding unhealthy habits such as smoking and overindulging in alcohol, and working to keep a healthy posture will help individually and together in reducing the pain you feel[42].

Avoiding stress if you can is important as when we're stressed our muscles remain tense for long periods causing tiredness, stiffness, pain and discomfort. Stress management, therefore, is an important part of pain management. Good sleep is necessary for any pain treatment to succeed and if you're not sleeping please speak to your doctor so that you can discuss the possibility of taking something to help you sleep at night.

You also have to be on the lookout for triggers that bring on your pain or worsen it, triggers such as overexertion, tiredness, staying in an uncomfortable position for any length of time, especially at night, overzealous gardening and strenuous household chores.

Chronic pain can have a profound effect on your mood and your mental state. You may find your self-esteem starts to dwindle, you have difficulty concentrating, your mood seems to swing from elation to feeling pessimistic much of the time. If this happens, you must consult your doctor.

Physical therapies are helpful in the management of chronic pain so hot and cold packs, massage, hydrotherapy, and daily exercise

---

42 https://jamanetwork.com/journals/jamanetworkopen/fullarticle/2828920?utm_source=For_The_Media&utm_medium=referral&utm_campaign=ftm_links&utm_term=011025

help most people to manage their pain. In addition, therapies such as CBT (cognitive behaviour therapy), relaxation exercises of all kinds, especially visualisation, meditation, mindfulness and acupuncture may be worth considering.

There are some natural remedies you might like to try, though I can't recommend them generally as there's no proof of effectiveness. Something like ginger root tea, or ginger oil rubbed in, topical capsaicin, yoga, stretches, may help your pain. For some people, cannabis provides powerful pain relief, particularly where there's muscle spasm so you should discuss this with your doctor as well. Don't be surprised if your doctor suggests that you might like to try a dose of an antidepressant to help with your pain. We know that some of the older antidepressants like amitriptyline can bring pain relief by helping us to think of pain in a different way.

Parkinson's Disease

PARKINSON'S DISEASE, LIKE DEMENTIA, IS a neurodegenerative disorder of the brain. The term, neurodegenerative means brain cells are killed off by disruptive proteins (dementia) or they simply die (Parkinson's disease). The cell death we see in Parkinson's has serious repercussions because the production of dopamine starts to shut down. Dopamine, once in the general circulation, is the chemical that keeps our muscle movements smooth, free-flowing, and coordinated. When it's not there our movements can become jerky, uncoordinated and muscles twitch. In Parkinson's disease one of the most notable symptoms is the tremor affecting the hands, plus the muscle stiffness that makes movements jerky and slow. Tremors of the hands and fingers are often the first sign and show up when a person is relaxed, but they may be able to control tremors to a certain degree when they concentrate on movements.

One of the tricks used by people suffering from Parkinson's disease is to hold a newspaper firmly. The tremor disappears when the grip is tightened by tensing muscles. Parkinson's shows in the face too which is classically mask-like with few facial expressions, and walking becomes a rapid shuffling movement with the body bent forward at the waist and the arms firmly by the side. When someone with Parkinson's walks the arms don't swing. The facial skin tends to be oily and there may be excess saliva.

Fortunately, we have medical and surgical treatments for Parkinson's disease. L-dopa makes up for lost dopamine and it's particularly good for movement, going part of the way to relieving tremor and difficulties with movement due to muscle stiffness. L-dopa is not a cure. Nor is surgery but it can often control some of the most troublesome physical symptoms. In surgery a patient is anesthetised and a probe put into the brain itself to localise an area that's causing tremor and then it's microscopically destroyed. This kind of surgery is getting more and more sophisticated and safer. There's a lot of research going on to improve it.

Besides medical and surgical treatments, there are physical treatments like physiotherapy, and occupational therapy providing an important background to any other kind of treatment.

Pedicures

IF YOU'VE NEVER HAD A pedicure in your life it's worth thinking about it going into your 60s, 70s and beyond. Our feet are always important to us but as we get older with calluses, corns and bunions, we're conscious of our feet as never before. It's worth taking care of them and a pedicure will go a long way to doing that. You're also in for a great treat.

A pedicure is like a facelift for the feet so put yourself in the hands of a pedicure expert who can often be found in a hairdressing salon or a nail bar. The dry, rough skin will be softened in a foot bath and removed where necessary. Your cracked heels will be gently dealt with, and a lot of thick skin removed. The gentle scrubbing renews and smooths the surface of your feet. A pedicure is finished off with nail varnish to your toenails. This might be a new sensation for you but really it's good fun, good for your morale too to see that you have young looking feet and cool toenails.

Your feet are the furthest distance from your heart. They're at the end of the line for their blood supply so it's easy for cuts and bruises to become infected and take a long time to heal. This is particularly important for diabetics because sugar levels in every part of their body, including their feet, are higher than normal. If there's any kind of an injury, even a tiny one, bacteria can enter the body through the skin, thrive and spread in your tissues making any infection worse. Regular pedicures are a necessity for anyone who has diabetes. If you do develop skin problems on your feet, consult your doctor or your pharmacist immediately so that you can get treatment to prevent a serious infection. An ulcer on your foot that doesn't heal must be examined by a doctor ASAP.

Keeping your feet in good nick

- Always wash your feet with pH-balanced soap, between your toes too. Dry them completely so moisture doesn't soften your skin leading to a fungus infection like athlete's foot.
- Inspect your feet every day for any redness, open skin sores, blisters, and ask your pharmacist for remedies. Pay attention to any sores that don't seem to heal or if you have numbness in your feet. See your GP ASAP.

- Visit a chiropodist (podiatrist) for corns and hard skin build-up. Wear "moisturising" socks at night.
- Change your socks every day. If your feet are prone to sweating change them more often. You could try an antiperspirant.
- Choose shoes that fit well so your toes aren't squashed and support your ankles.
- Don't forget to moisturise. The skin on your feet can get very dry and cracked causing painful sores. Use a rich lotion or foot cream every day.
- Work your feet. Moving your feet in a circular motion, standing on your toes, flexing your feet towards you can all help with your circulation and to avoid joint pain and other issues.

Pets

I'VE BEEN WAVERING ABOUT GETTING a dog. We always had a dog in the family when I was a child. We had dogs when my children were growing up. I confess, I yearn for a dog to see me through my last years. So why am I hesitating? Well, a dog is a responsibility. As I travel a bit, I'm loath to leave my dog alone. It's not fair. Even if I'm prepared to take the dog with me, travelling with a dog isn't easy. For instance, Eurostar doesn't allow dogs on their trains and most budget airlines don't allow dogs on their planes except if they're "assistance dogs". The answer seems to be trains and cars, though a journey from London to Toulouse, one which I undertake quite often, would be challenging.

Would family look after my dog, or a kind friend? And what about the toilet training if I opt for a puppy? It would be difficult for me to get down on my knees to mop up accidents, and then get up again! And what about the necessary early morning walks and walks last thing at night, in all weathers? Am I up to it? Do I want my life reordered in this way? Then there are the expenses such as vet fees, pet insurance, accessories. Am I prepared to do all this for doggy companionship? And most importantly, who would look after my dog when I die? I couldn't contemplate getting a dog without knowing this, but now I do so I've taken the plunge and I'm getting a dog. My black Labrador puppy called Alfie is staying with the breeder to be fully trained then he'll be mine.

There are upsides, of course – the companionship, the daily exercise (in all weathers), loyalty and unconditional love. There are other doggy skills from which I might benefit. Dogs can smell when diabetes is coming on, that is prediabetes, which might send you to your doctor for early assessment. They also can smell cancer. We know that dogs are good for the health and happiness of old people. I recall an experiment where the blood pressure of hospital patients was tracked, and over 300 different factors were taken into consideration. The only thing that lowered blood pressure reliably was found to be stroking a dog. There you have it. We also know that dogs are good for the mental health of people who are living in care homes. Just seeing them appears to be enough to make them smile and raise their mood.

How to choose a dog

Having said that, there are several factors you should consider when choosing a dog:
- Do you have a garden or do you live in a flat?
- What size of dog do you want?
- Do you want a puppy or a trained adult dog?
- Pure-breed or cross-breed?
- From a breeder or a shelter? If from a breeder, how much money do you want to spend?

- Do you have allergies and need to consider hypoallergenic dogs?
- What features do you prefer in a dog?
- How would the dog fit into your lifestyle?
- What are the legal requirements?
- What happens to your dog when you die?

You may not be a dog person but there are many other animals to choose from that could be a pet for you. Make sure you weigh up the pros and cons before choosing an animal companion because a pet is for life.

Posture

MOST OF US HAVE CHILDHOOD memories of being encouraged to have good posture by a teacher going along a row of desks punching each child in the back to discourage round shoulders. Well, posture is much more important than that, especially as you get older. It has so many pay offs and bonuses. First of all, if you gently pull in your tummy, lift up your back, lower your shoulders and pull your chin down and back so you look straight ahead, your silhouette is automatically taller and neater. You look 10 pounds lighter.

That's an instant improvement and other benefits accrue if you become posture-conscious. Good posture relieves back ache and stops shoulder and neck pain. We have a chain of bones, joints and muscles that extends from our heels up to the knees and hips, ascending through the pelvis to the spine right up to the neck and the skull. It's called the spinal chain. This chain is very happy if we keep all the elements in line through good posture.

You get all these benefits if you keep your head and neck in line with your spine. What this alignment does is to keep your weight running in a straight line downwards from head to toe. When this happens your body becomes weightless so muscles are in neutral and relaxed. There's no stress on joints which otherwise would have to strain to keep your body upright. Your very heavy head is held in line with your neck and your spinal muscles don't become tired and achy, supporting and protecting your spine. Your stretched muscles can rest.

If, however, the spinal chain is disrupted by arthritis, a slipped disc, muscle strain and bad posture, the chain is deformed, the result being headaches, neck and shoulder pain, lower back pain and sciatica.

Importance of your core

For all this to happen and your spinal chain to be aligned you have to "put on your core". This refers to contracting your abdominal muscles and your erector spinae muscles of your lower back. When you put these muscles "on" (pull them in) they form a strong corset around your body that holds up your spine and rests the overworked muscles of your back. You can give your lower back instant relief by recruiting these strong muscles to ease, strengthen and protect your back, and you can do this anytime, anywhere. First, pull your tummy muscles inwards and upwards towards your back. Then elongate your back from your hips to your ribs. Now your muscular corset is in place and you have instant relief from backache. Quite a trick.

Your core is crucial to keep you free of pain from overstretched muscle. It's worth giving them daily attention, pulling in your abdominals whenever you remember and if you feel up to it, doing a few gentle planks and press-ups two to three times a week for 20 minutes. And pull in your abs every few minutes when you're walking.

Looking after your spine

As we get on we find ourselves spending more and more time sitting and this isn't good for your spine. It can bring on back pain. Around one in five people suffer from it. If you have back pain these suggestions might help:

- Quit smoking. Why? Smoking, high blood pressure and coronary artery disease are linked to low back pain.
- Your spine is the happiest when it's straight so adjust your posture to keep it straight. It's easy to slouch if we sit for a long time and stare at a computer screen. Every half an hour, get up and walk around.
- Having strong and supple core muscles will help alleviate the pain so keep exercising and lose some weight.
- Increase the amount of fruit, vegetables, lean meat, fish and wholegrains you eat.

How to spend less time sitting

We all live increasingly sedentary lives, yet there's plenty of research saying sitting for too long isn't good for us. Did you know the over 65s spend 10 hours or more each day sitting or lying down, making them the most sedentary population group. Sitting for too long is bad for your health, regardless of how much exercise you do.

So here are some tips to help you get out that easy chair:

- Stand up and move during TV ad breaks.
- Use the stairs as much as possible.
- Set a reminder to get up every 30 minutes and walk around for a couple of minutes.
- Alternate working seated with working standing.
- Do most types of your own housework.

- Place a laptop on a box or similar to work standing. I've got a special table top stand for my laptop so I stand to do all my work on a computer.
- Stand and walk around while on the phone.
- Take a walk every time you get a coffee or tea.
- Walk to a colleague's desk instead of emailing or calling.
- Swap some TV time for active hobbies such as gardening and DIY.
- Join in community-based activities, such as dance classes and walking groups.
- Join in active play with the grandchildren.

Prostate Gland

YOUR PROSTATE GLAND NESTLES AROUND the base of your bladder, circling the urethra, the tube that carries urine to your penis and to the outside. Its job is to make a nutritious fluid that keeps sperm healthy and strong. Over time it has a tendency to become enlarged, as in BPH (benign prostatic hypertrophy), and if part of the gland protrudes into the urethra, it will cut down the flow of urine and lead to symptoms like dribbling, difficulty in starting the flow of urine, urgency to empty the bladder and a poor stream. Because the enlarged prostate irritates the urethra, men with BPH often have to get up in the night to pass urine. Both BPH and early prostatic cancer have similar symptoms and are easy to treat if caught early. Any man who has prostatic symptoms should have them checked out as soon as possible by his doctor. This way a cancer of the prostate would be caught early when it can be cured.

Prostate cancer screening

This is important for all men over the age of 50 as it's the second biggest cancer killer of men. It may be silent until it's quite advanced but the possibility of detecting it early has been simplified by a blood test for a chemical marker for prostate disease, the prostate specific antigen, or PSA. However, it has a tendency to give false positives.

The good news is that other tools for cancer screening are being investigated and the latest is a simple saliva test, though what the test looks for is highly sophisticated. It locates over 130 gene variants linked to prostate cancer and has proven to be accurate. Importantly, it can indicate if the cancer is slow or fast-growing and so plays an important part in determining treatment. It could turn the tide on prostate cancer. In the meantime, there is the urine test MPS2 and genetic biomarkers such as PH1 and PCA3. It's hoped that those more sensitive tests will result in less radical surgery to remove the gland in its entirety when that's not necessary and more "watchful waiting" of a cancer that initially grows slowly. Before your cancer surgery make sure you have a full discussion with your surgeon about the possibility of side effects including difficulty getting an erection.

How you can lower your prostate cancer risk

It's not possible to give precise suggestions as to how you can lower your risk of any cancer because I don't know your medical details. But I can tell you about lifestyle factors that might lower your risk.

These lifestyle factors will PROBABLY help protect you:
- Eat less meat, milk and other dairy products.
- Eat less saturated fats.
- Soya products are good and tomatoes (for lycopene, an anti-prostate cancer chemical), vegetables.
- Eat more foods containing yellow/orange carotenoids

(carrots, sweet potatoes, cantaloupes), flavonoids (berries, citrus fruits, kale, apple), vitamins D (oily fish like salmon, mackerel, and sardines, egg yolks and liver) and vitamin E (nuts, seeds, vegetable oils, spinach, broccoli).

And these may POSSIBLY help too:
- Eat fewer calories.
- Drink less alcohol.
- Keep your weight in check.
- Eat more polyunsaturated fatty acids from vegetables e.g. nuts, seeds, avocado.

Treatment

The treatment for your prostate cancer will depend on how long you've had it, its aggressiveness, and the opinions of your doctors. If investigations reveal that you have a very slow growing cancer your doctors may recommend a regime of "watch and wait" with frequent check ups on its progress. Treatments often are combinations of surgery, chemotherapy, x-ray therapy, immunotherapy and hormone therapy. Your oncologist, in collaboration with you, will decide on a plan of which treatments are to be used to best treat your cancer.

Protein

I'M INCLUDING A SPECIAL MENTION of protein separately from other foods for several reasons. First of all protein often contains essential vitamins and minerals, one of them being iron which we need to prevent anaemia. Red meat is the most efficient food package of iron so to keep your iron stores topped up you only need to eat a few ounces (70g) of red meat a couple of times a week. Make sure you eat some vitamin C (veg, tomatoes, fresh peppers) with it as it helps your body to absorb iron. Dark green leaves will give you iron too, with vitamin C built in. Our culture warns against eating too much red meat for good reasons but don't abandon it, it's such a convenient way to get your iron. Trouble is we tend to eat less and less protein as we get older.

Protein is filling so we can't eat a whole steak the way we used to but we do need it for our muscles, bones, joints, hair and skin to help keep them in good repair and to promote healing when they're injured. Fortunately, there's more than one kind of protein, divided basically into those derived from animals and those derived from plants. Not for nothing were these called first class and second class proteins. Animal protein (first class) provides you with all the body's building blocks (amino acids) you need whereas plants (second class) are short of some amino acids, so if you're a vegetarian you have to eat a great variety of plants in large quantities to get what you need. You could also eat foods fortified by vitamins such as cereals and bread.

Another reason for making sure you eat enough protein, first of all animal protein e.g. meat, fish, eggs, dairy and secondly plant protein e.g. lentils, peas, beans (especially soya beans), sweetcorn, chickpeas, nuts, seeds, quinoa, is because we lose a lot of protein as we age through shrinking muscles.

Age-related loss of muscle mass can begin when someone is in their 40s. By their 60s, people start losing muscle mass on average around 1% per year. You can slow it down with various exercises such as weight training but muscle mass will only increase if the exercises you do become harder. This loss of muscle is most noticeable in our large muscles of the legs, arms and torso, where it's responsible for strength, stamina and coordination.

Adults need 0.75g of protein per kg of body weight per day[43], so for someone who's 70kg (11st) that's 52.5g (2 eggs + a 100g steak or 150g lentils + 150g of chicken). A good measure of a protein portion is the palm of your hand e.g. a handful of nuts. So in order to get protein into your diet you could have eggs for breakfast, a mid-morning snack of nuts, and for lunch salmon or tuna, out of a tin if that's all you have.

Eating protein can help you lose weight. Here's how:

If you eat 2,000 calories a day, up your protein intake to 50-175 grams, that's 10%-35% of your daily calories. Your body burns more calories digesting protein than carbohydrates, so just by eating protein, you're already burning more calories.

But what if you're going short of calories? Here are a few high-calorie healthy nutritious foods: nuts, avocado, bananas, oily fish, eggs, dark chocolate, potatoes and quinoa.

And if you're worried you're eating too much red meat here are a few suggestions how you can start eating less.

How to eat less red meat

- Concentrate on **vegetables** and eat them first then you'll have less room for meat.
- Sip **water** while you eat and you'll feel sated sooner.
- A **tuna sandwich** can be as delicious as beef or chicken.
- **Seafood** is great, substitute it for red meat. I'd forgotten about shellfish which I love and now eat crab and prawns each week.
- Try **grilled salmon** and other dark-fleshed fish like tuna and trout instead of beef.
- Try vegetarian sausages or soya bacon bits on your pizza.

---

[43] https://www.bhf.org.uk/informationsupport/heart-matters-magazine/nutrition/protein#:~:text=Most%20adults%20need%20around%200.75,the%20palm%20of%20your%20hand

- **Don't go cold turkey,** be easy on yourself and gradually reduce the amount of red meat you eat.
- Try substituting a **tofu burger** for a hamburger.
- As a rule of thumb the amount of meat you eat with a meal shouldn't be bigger than the palm of your hand.
- Fish and shellfish are easy to barbeque, try **trout, salmon or tuna** seasoned with herbs – barbecued fish is delicious.

Pulse

How to take your pulse

Knowing how and where to take your own pulse is wise at any time but as we get older it's a skill that we really should acquire. Personally, I reach for my pulse whenever I feel dizzy or very tired just to make sure it's regular and my heart is doing its job. Taking your pulse is a really useful backstop. It means at any point you can make a quick assessment of what's not quite right and whether you need a doctor.

What is your pulse?

Every time your heart beats it pumps out blood that circulates round the body. That pumping action results in a wave of pressure each time the heart beats. That can be felt wherever an artery lies close to the surface of your skin. Because an artery can be felt easily on the underside of your wrist in line with your thumb that's where we tend to take our pulse. You can, however, also feel your pulse in your neck, this is the carotid pulse and up the arch of the foot in line with the big toe, and in the centre of your groin. Basically, your pulse rate is your heart rate.

How do you feel for your pulse?

On the underside of your left wrist and in line with your left thumb feel for the pulse with the tips of the first three fingers of your right hand. Count the number of beats you can feel in 15 seconds and multiply by four to get the rate per minute. A normal resting pulse is regular and strong and the average rate is 72/minute but can be anything between 60-100. People who are fit like athletes tend to have a lower than normal heart rate.

What you might discover when you take your pulse

Your pulse isn't regular all the time. You may find your pulse rate increases as you breathe in and as you breathe out it slows down. Don't worry, this is a normal variation in the pulse rate brought about by breathing. If this happens, wait for a few minutes and start taking your pulse again breathing normally in and out as you take your pulse.
Your pulse seems to miss a beat. This can also be normal but see your doctor if you're concerned.
Your pulse is irregular. This probably means you have an arrhythmia and your heart is beating irregularly. It's not always an emergency and if you feel okay, consult your doctor as soon as possible. If, on the other hand, you're feeling breathless or you have chest pain you should call an ambulance immediately because this kind of irregularity, atrial fibrillation (AF), needs full assessment and treatment with specific drugs.

Exercise keeps your heart strong

Exercise that makes you breathe faster (aerobic exercise) will keep your heart healthy. We now know short bursts of this kind of exercise that ups your heart rate for as little as a few minutes, boosts heart health.

Your target heart rate (HR) is the heart rate achieved through exercise that's necessary for heart health. It varies with age so here's a table of ages and appropriate heart rates as estimated by the American Heart Association (www.heart.org) which I've simplified for you.

Age (years)	Target HR	Maximum HR
20	100-170 bpm	200 bpm
30	95-162 bpm	190 bpm
35	93-157 bpm	185 bpm
40	90-153 bpm	180 bpm
45	88-149 bpm	175 bpm
50	85-145 bpm	170 bpm
55	83-140 bpm	165 bpm
60	80-136 bpm	160 bpm
65	78-132 bpm	155 bpm
70	75-128 bpm	150 bpm
75	73-123 bpm	145 bpm
80	70-119 bpm	140 bpm
85	68-113 bpm	135 bpm
90	65-111 bpm	130 bpm

Q

Quads – The Importance Of

YOUR QUADS, THOSE HUGE MUSCLES on the front of your thighs, are important all through your life for walking, running, cycling and jumping, but particularly so as we get older. The simple reason is they get you out of a chair from sitting to standing. You can see why that's so important. If your quads are weak you're imprisoned in your chair, unable to get out of it and you won't be able to walk. You'll find yourself sitting for hours on end and we know that's not good. It's not just that your quads will get weaker, as the biggest muscles in the body, they put the heart and lungs through their paces because every time you use them they need more oxygen. So it's worth keeping your quads in good nick all your life.

To prevent losing muscle mass you can exercise your quads with cycling, jogging, running and walking. But you don't even have to leave home to exercise your quads. All you need is a chair. And all you have to do is to raise yourself out of it 14-15 times once a day using your thighs, with your hands crossed on your chest. Your quads can keep you engaged with life, not on the sidelines. They're there to help you stay active and to help strengthen your back.

Don't find yourself at 70 or 80 operating at the limit of your physical powers. Quads are crucial for your balance and therefore for your confidence to be mobile, flexible and agile. Without strong quads you're more likely to fall and sustain a fracture which, if you have osteoporosis, may take a long time to knit.

Exercising your quads

- Just stand. The great benefit of standing is that the weight of your whole body is pulling down on your skeleton. This doesn't only help to keep your bones strong, it tones up your muscles, some of them the biggest muscles in the body like your quads on the front of your thighs and your hamstrings on the back. And, if you stand in a good posture it improves your core strength.
- Squats are great to keep your thighs (quads) and buttocks (glutes) in good shape. It's like sitting down on a chair without using your arms. If you're a bit unsteady try squats on a chair with the seat at knee level but instead of sitting down just touch your bottom to the seat then stand up. Start with five reps then increase them.
- Getting around on your bike builds leg strength. Pedalling tones your quads and hamstrings as well as your calves.
- Single-leg squats are perfect for working your quads and hips. Stand upright with hands on hips and raise your left foot. Hinge forward slightly as you bend the right knee and carefully lower down without it collapsing inwards. Try to get a bit lower each week. Hang on to something if your balance isn't good.

R

Reading

I COULDN'T LIVE WITHOUT READING. I'M inclined to fill moments during the day by reaching for something to read, starting soon after I wake with the newspaper. I usually have a book or two on the go as I like reading more than one at a time. I've always found not having something to read makes me nervous. I get anxious if I'm not carrying something with me that I can dip into if I have a few free moments. I've often wondered what I find so appealing about reading. I've found I'm not only attracted to reading, it's often reassuring and deeply satisfying, satisfying in a way I didn't recognise in the beginning. It's one of the ways I use to control any anxiety I might be feeling at the time. Reading calms my mind and gives me a more positive view of life. It fills my mind so there's no room for intrusive, negative thoughts. I guess I use reading as therapy and to keep my "naughty little amygdala" – the centre of the brain that causes anxiety – under control.

When I find myself in certain situations without a book or a newspaper I'll read practically anything, pamphlets, brochures, even the ingredients list on a bottle of sauce. So in a way, I use reading to control not only my head but to control my world if I feel it's getting the better of me. Reading orders the world and makes sense of life. Three of my favourite authors are guaranteed to make sense of the imponderables in life. Two of them are women and there's one man. I was so fond of Iris Murdoch that I would find out the date of publication of every new novel and order it from the bookshop so that I could start reading it immediately. As well as being a writer, Iris Murdoch was a philosopher working at Cambridge University and her novels are full of people living very complicated lives. I remember once finding myself in an eccentric situation and thinking, "Gosh. This is like being in an Iris Murdoch novel."

About the same time I first read Margaret Atwood. She set me back on my heels. She was one of the first feminist voices that I "heard". Not a raucous voice but a modulated, reasonable, rational voice pointing out the injustices of a male-dominated society. She deflates pomposity and cruelty with humour and sarcasm. I remember the joy at first reading her novels because I thought, "at last someone agrees with me." And I laughed. Margaret Atwood so reliably examines our world and the place of women in it that I sought out every new book she published. Third on my list is Philip Roth and when I finished one of his novels, I would pine for the next. Roth is quite different from the two women. He was a classical New Yorker and someone I would describe as rough. By that I mean he's unafraid to express controversial ideas and to stand by them, something I greatly admire. He shines a light not just on New York life but New York family life in much the same way as Arthur Miller. On the surface, Roth appears to be a simple storyteller, but he's not. He's a very deep thinker reflecting on a world view, as well as an American view and a family view.

I discovered only in the last few years a fourth, Annie Ernaux, a French woman who, from the beginning of her teenage years, has been a feminist. She wrote about her life and how her feminist ideas often clashed with what was happening to her. Her writing is harrowing, always honest, and always painful. She has won the Nobel Prize for Literature and I've read everything she's ever written. I find her a great comfort because she speaks directly to me from the page. I'm just getting into Han Kang, a South Korean writer. At this point I've only read one of her novels, *The Vegetarian*, which won her the International Booker Prize. It describes how a beautiful young woman wrests control of her repressive life by refusing to eat meat – something unheard of in her culture. And just a few months ago I started to read Claire Keegan, a writer in the great Irish tradition, pithy, poetic and heart-wrenching.

Thank heavens there are always books to read.

Remarriage & New Partnerships

I REMEMBER ONCE BEING ON THE platform with Princess Diana at a charity do. In my speech I mentioned I thought marriage should come with a government health warning. I heard her laughing heartily behind me and later she took me aside and said, giggling, my recommendation that marriage should be accompanied by a health warning should be better known. Little did we know...

In a general sense, as you might suspect, men are healthier in marriage than women. For instance, married women have higher hospital admission rates than married men. Remarriage is quicker and more common in widowers than it is in widows. This is especially so if widowers have left behind a happy marriage. After years of a loving relationship and companionship they begin to miss home comforts. Many women don't feel the same. They're cognisant that marrying an older man may mean a problematical future if she has to look after a man with heart disease, diabetes, high blood pressure and mobility issues. In straightened circumstances a woman may hesitate to embark on a new long-term relationship because she's possessive about her assets, her salary and her alimony, all of which she might want to protect as a nest egg against the future. In this situation, a little self-examination doesn't go amiss. Think about the kind of person you are and what you really would like to get out of the years left to you. If contemplating remarriage it may be helpful to ask yourself if you can trust your prospective partner with everything that's yours. It would be a mistake to marry if you don't.

If you're both retired, there's another important consideration. You're going to be spending 24 hours a day together. This may not be what you're used to. If your partner went to work from nine to five and you've enjoyed having the home to yourself, living together may be a source of friction and conflict. So make sure you map out your days together before you commit yourself.

You may have sought a new partnership and remarried because it's important to you to have a long-standing, loving relationship in old age. And I agree with you. Sex may not be the priority, but loving companionship is, because it's so life-affirming for you both and brings reassurance that you're still a desirable person who can make another person happy. That's a great comfort as you get older. Mind you, sex isn't to be completely relegated because older people who have an active sex life, albeit less frequently than they used to in their younger days, have more confidence and self-esteem than those who choose to be celibate.

One of the aspects of having a partner that isn't often talked about is they can act as a gate keeper between you and the outside world. With a partner, you can feel it's us against the rest of the world. That's precious and life-affirming. Loving partners can reassure each other that their emotional needs are recognised and acknowledged. It's reassuring to know that you can absolutely be yourself with another person and not hold back. Most older people don't feel that they have to conform to the rules laid down by society. They feel they have lived long enough to ignore the criticism of others and can please themselves.

Resting

WHEN I WAS A TEENAGER, my mum used to say I worked hard and I played hard. Now that I'm in my late 80s, neither of these things apply to me anymore. I would paraphrase her words as "walk hard, rest hard". Since about my 50s I've always given consideration to resting my body after it's been physically challenged. My husband used to do what he called the Horizon Walk in the Black Mountains in Wales, about 25 miles. I did it with him once. Only once. Because I had to rest up for three whole days for my body to recover.

Trekking in the Himalayas in my early 50s almost broke my body and I think this was because there was no opportunity for resting. After a day's trekking, we would go to bed around 8pm but we were up at 5am to continue trekking, and my tiredness accumulated. When I got back to the UK I had to "rest" my body for almost six weeks before it got back to normal.

I perceive resting as an important part of staying fit. After vigorous exercise, the body needs to recover and the older we get, the longer that takes, so it pays to be sensitive to your rest needs. I've never seen resting in bed as laziness but as a necessity to allow my body to refresh itself. These days if I do a walk of more than two miles I stay in bed till lunchtime on the following day, and the day after that if need be.

What's going on in your body during rest and recovery is the minor tears that occur in muscles when you're exercising hard are repairing themselves. The muscles are also getting rid of waste products from burning the energy they used during exercise. A good illustration of this is muscles which have been exercised hard and need to get rid of lactic acid which has accumulated in them because the exercise outstripped their oxygen supply. You can see this happening before your eyes if you watch an interview on television with an athlete who's just completed a very strenuous event, let's say the 800 metres. They're being interviewed several minutes after the completion of the event, but they're still panting because the muscles are continuing to get rid of lactic acid which has accumulated during "anaerobic" exercise.

Retirement

RETIREMENT, EVEN IF YOU PREPARE for it carefully, can be a stressful time. It's not surprising given almost overnight you have to cope with loss of a job which may have been your major source of interest and self-worth, loss of contact with colleagues and workmates, plus a fall in income. Don't let it make you think your useful life has ended. It hasn't. The root of the problem is nearly always difficulty in facing up to change. That may lead to doubting yourself, even considering yourself worthless. It's tough for anyone to keep their spirits up if they feel they're a liability and find stopping work hard. You needn't feel this way.

Retirement can be the beginning of renewal and fresh interests, especially those with family, friends and neighbours. You have so much time on your hands to devote to new activities and relationships. Furthermore, these late relationships may turn out to be rewarding because they're special and more personal. See retirement as an opportunity to explore the company of others and join in groups of new friends[44].

What often scares us is the prospect of retirement rather than retirement itself. Given reasonable health and sufficient income, a retired man or woman soon adapts to the change in their life and both their outlook and physical health improve. All of us have to adjust to retirement and some of us do it better than others. I doubt I'll ever retire, I like working too much. To enjoy retirement, however, we need to prepare for it and plan for the long-term. Not preparing soon enough and being caught without essentials in place inevitably causes anxiety.

Preparation comes down to putting money aside, buying and disposing of personal property and assets, getting advice about inheritance tax (IHT), attending to health needs, getting information and advice about leisure time interests, and generally changing the balance between working and your new life. Good preparation means looking after income and assets to provide for your life when retired.

Some continuation of earlier working activities or social relationships can promote a sense of belonging and still being useful. There's some early research in very old Japanese men who continued to go into work for as little as half a day a week. They were healthier and happier than men who didn't. This research is old but it's very interesting. Paying attention to health and physical comforts will make room for more activity and security, up your sense of achievement, usefulness and happiness.

Here are some thoughts about enjoying retirement

Generally women find retirement easier than men. As a woman, you've probably stayed in touch with your family and friends where

---

44   https://mensline.org.au/mens-mental-health/adjusting-to-retirement/

you have status so you know you're loved and respected. A man, however, may see his job and his earning capacity as important status symbols and finds retirement a blow when they suddenly disappear.

About six months before you retire try living on your retirement income. It could be more straightforward than you imagined and you'll also see where you need to make savings.

Plan carefully, ahead of retirement, (even several years ahead), paying attention to your financial arrangements, housing, healthcare as well as socialising, hobbies, interests and activities you plan to continue when you're retired.

When one partner stops work and the other continues, have a heart to heart before accepting your days will be out of sync. Assess the problem and work out possible solutions. Together make a plan that suits both of you including weekends, and stick to that plan.

Spend all you can on advice to make your money work for you. Draw up a budget even if you've never done it before. Your bank manager or an accountant can help you with the details.

A rota for the household chores is essential or resentment may build, especially if you've never shared before.

Delve into the past and see people you've lost touch with and who you'd like to see again.

Rather than feeling left alone, you could start new projects and take up old interests, remembering old passions and renewing them.

Both partners in a relationship should be prepared to give and take when approaching the adjustments retirement demands.

Do pamper yourself if you've got lots of spare time. Arrange rounds of golf with your mates. Have your hair done, arrange a pedicure, sleep late, read in the afternoon, go see a movie and put your feet up whenever you feel like it. Because you're worth it!

Sex, Drugs & Walking Sticks

If you find yourself at home with lots of time on your hands, talk to your partner about how best to spend your leisure time together.

S

Sex... It Never Stops

I CAN SAY THIS FROM THE perspective of great age, we'll be very glad when we're old that we kept sex alive in middle age. Why? Well, a couple who's got into the habit of sharing physical affection over a lifetime will continue to share cuddles as they get older whereas a couple who lost the habit of caressing each other in middle age won't. I've thought for a long time the frequency of sex means less and less as we get older. Frequency, of itself, doesn't enrich. Meaningful sex does, even if it's only once a month. It's imbued with a lifetime of loving and captures the feeling of being desirable and sexually alive.

Introduce yourself to the thought that sex isn't the only way to love. Sex is only one of the myriad ways of loving. It certainly helps if you and your partner deescalate penetrative sex and orgasm so you can focus on pleasing your partner with caring and sharing. There's a lot to be said for platonic relationships when people are brought together by a common purpose. There can be deep, fulfilling and satisfying love. Just think of office romances, often passionate and lustful, where two people are devoted not just to each other but to a common goal. But for many people sex remains an important part of love.

There's nothing to fear about sex in our older years if we believe, as I do, that our evolution as sexual beings continues till we die.

That evolution takes us through several sexual stages or sexual milestones as we pass from our lusty 40s, to our adventurous 50s, onto our vibrant 60s and thence to our loving 70s, 80s and 90s with a lifetime partner, or with someone new. Truth is we don't feel very different inside about love as we get older. Our passion and tenderness don't desert us. We can feel as sexually attracted to someone as we ever did. For sure we never lose the desire to love and be loved. If anything, as we get older there are more ways to express our sexuality than ever because we're free of inhibitions and ossified social customs.

Some recent research has shown that staying fit in your middle years pays off in your 60s and 70s so if you want to be fit enough to enjoy sex in your later years, keep fit and healthy in your 40s and 50s[45]. We soon discover being unfit puts the brakes on sex and may even rule it out. Spontaneous sex is certainly difficult if either of you has a chronic illness affecting the lungs, heart, muscle strength and joints. It would be sad to miss out on sex for want of a fit, healthy, agile body as we get older.

Some good news about our sexuality as we grow older

Well, honestly, all the news about sexuality as we get on is good. Quite a bit of research in older people confirms the sex drive, enjoyment and pleasure of sex are, if anything, greater than in younger years[46]. And that's cause for celebration because sex, at any age, makes us feel attractive, appreciated and loved. It relieves tension by completely filling our minds.

In an English study, 86% of men and 60% of women aged 60-69

---

45   https://jamanetwork.com/journals/jamanetworkopen/fullarticle/2727269?utm_source=JAMA_Network&utm_medium=referral&utm_campaign=ftm_links&utm_term=030819

46   https://www.nia.nih.gov/health/sexuality/sexuality-and-intimacy-older-adults#:~:text=How%20you%20physically%20feel%20may,no%20worries%20about%20getting%20pregnant

were sexually active. Even more encouraging, 59% of men and 34% of women aged 70–79 were sexually active, and 31% of men and 14% of women 80 years or older. Even 10% of people over 90 years reported being still sexually active in a Swedish study. And if you're looking for more, in a US study of people aged 75-85 years who were sexually active, 54% reported having sex two or three times per month and 23% reported having sex one or more times per week[47]. But many people are happy with intimacy for its own sake. And many still relish non-penetrative sex including oral sex, kissing, fondling and solo sex – masturbation.

American researchers, Arthur Kinsey in the late 40s, Masters and Johnson in the late 50s and 60s and Shere Hite in the 70s painted positive pictures of sex for both women and men. And if you want more to cheer about, here it is from *The Starr-Weiner Report on Sex and Sexuality in the Mature Years* by Bernard D. Starr and Marcella Bakur Weiner published in 1982, but interesting nonetheless. Little has changed according to UK, Swedish and Polish studies.

- Oral sex is the most exciting part of sex for many people.
- During our 60s, 70s and 80s we're sexually active and that goes for most of us including widows, widowers, divorcees and singles.
- We're quite prepared to experiment for rewarding sex.
- Women and men consider masturbation a perfectly acceptable way to satisfy their sexual needs.
- Most women who had orgasms when they were young, still have them. Orgasm is an essential part of our sex lives and it may be stronger than in the past.
- We're no longer embarrassed or anxious about sex.

---

47   https://www.thelancet.com/journals/lanhl/article/PIIS2666-7568(23)00003-X/fulltext

- We don't crave a younger lover, someone near to our own age would be ideal.
- Losing inhibitions means most of us enjoy being naked when we have sex. Nudity isn't a problem.
- Our view of sex doesn't change as we get older and we think it'll be the same in the future.

On behalf of all women I want to pay tribute to Shere Hite. When I first read her research on sex in women, having spoken to hundreds of them, the scales fell from my eyes. She revealed information about our sexuality that had been suppressed for centuries by men peddling a male construct, denying us our sexuality. In her book, *The Hite Report*, she gave liberating news to all women. Here's a summary. A woman of 80 has the same physical potential for orgasm as she did at 20. Just as important is the fact that a woman's clitoris remains as responsive as ever, at least until the mid-70s, and I think beyond. The response from clitoral stimulation is the same in older women as it is in younger ones. I read her book and was immediately converted to her point of view of women as sexual beings. I felt I must be her standard bearer and from then on I tried to reverse the male view of women's sexuality and sexual pleasure by unpicking the lies women had been told for eons.

At any age a dry vagina can make penetration difficult and painful to the extent that it may rule out sexual intercourse altogether. A dry vagina can occur for all kinds of reasons at different ages. In a younger woman anxiety may be enough. Not being attracted to the person you're having sex with is also a reason. Then there's the menopause when a woman's oestrogen is more or less turned off like a tap. As the vagina relies for its health on oestrogen it stops producing lubrication, dries out and becomes thin, sore and vulnerable to infection. With the cooperation of her doctor a woman may safely use intravaginal oestrogen and, before sex, lubricate the entrance to her vagina with water based, pH-controlled vaginal gel, or ask her partner to do it for her.

Does our sexuality diminish over time?

Yes, it does, but why would we expect it not to? It's far better to concentrate on what we've got than be resentful and bitter about what we've lost. Changes due to age shouldn't surprise or depress you. Here are a few stats to prepare you.

Men in their 50-60s
Erections are fugitive and take longer to achieve and require more direct stimulation than before. It's less rigid but probably rigid enough to enter a partner's vagina should you both want.

With increasing age an erection subsides faster after ejaculation than before.

Ejaculation is different too. There's nearly always less semen than in the past and ejaculation lasts a shorter time with less force. Whereas when you were younger you could be ready for more sex in an hour or less, it's now longer before you can manage another erection, and an orgasm. This is called the "refractory period" and it gets longer and longer as you age. So it may be a week or longer in your 70s and 80s.

Women aged 51-78
Even with intravaginal oestrogen the vagina is less stretchy than in the past but this has been changing since the menopause.

During the 60s the clitoris begins to shrink but the wonderful thing is, it responds to stimulation and will continue to respond into your 80s, even 90s.

Arousal takes longer than when you were younger but you can speed it up with masturbation and a vibrator.

You needn't go short of orgasms as you get older as they tend to be more intense with age but they may be shorter.

In general, lubrication takes longer than before, that's where lubricating gels and jellies come in.

These findings are averages of many women so they don't apply to individual women. In that sense they don't apply specifically to you. They're simply general statements, but interesting nonetheless, of what starts to happen as we get older so you can take changes in your stride.

Erections, Erectile Disfunction (ED)

Sadly, the news isn't as good for men. Such is the mystique surrounding erections, getting them and maintaining them, it comes as no surprise that a man, faced with erectile dysfunction, feels his sex life is over. And of course his impotence is not just his business but also his partner's and the business of their relationship.

Despite the challenge of impotence it would be wrong to think that a couple's sex life is over. Rather than descending into an aversion for sex and avoiding it, it's the time to talk, to be open, and look for new options together. And there are plenty of options.

Even if this happens repeatedly there's no need for a man to think of himself as impotent. A man may have sustained damage to his penile nerves which are necessary to get an erection. Mind you ED needn't be due to age alone. Indeed most 17-year-olds have experienced it. Fear on its own can sometimes be enough. And when fear turns to dread, an erection is well nigh impossible.

Heart disease is always worrying and a man who's had a heart attack may recoil from sex thinking the strenuous exercise could precipitate another. Consult your doctor and I'm sure they'll reassure you, as long as you take it easy.

The good news is that older men can take advantage of any of the treatments used for ED. You should know that the success of therapies is encouraging and definitely worth a try. It helps if you're prepared to make a few adjustments.

Concerns about erection

Some men think they're not a real man if their erection is no longer reliable. They're letting their partner down. They worry about it and what their partner might think. You may be surprised to hear most women understand, and it would be wrong to give yourself a hard time. Anxiety alone can compromise an erection. The solution is to talk together and work at finding a new kind of sex. Knowing how an erection works and what might cause it to go wrong will illuminate the problem and give you both a fresh perspective. I think it would help both men and women to know how an erection happens because I believe a greater comprehension of an erection's mechanism would enlighten both partners, make for mutual understanding and dissipate any resentment.

How an erection works

When we blow up a balloon with air it becomes bigger, stretched and tight. The stiffness of an erection depends on blood filling specially designed spaces in the penis (the corpus cavernosum) and stretching them making the penis turgid. That's only stage one. To maintain an erection that blood can't be allowed to drain away. To keep it in the penis special valves in the corpus cavernosum snap shut and trap the blood in the penis.

Unsurprisingly the brain is involved through connections to the penile nerves which run down the side of the penis and control erections. So there's the explanation of a man seeing a sexual image and a split second later the blood starts to pump. He feels his erection begin. It's called the brain-penis connection.

And its importance can't be overemphasised because any interference with that connection, like damage to the penile nerves as in diabetes and furring up of the penile arteries as with high blood pressure, can mean insufficient blood getting into the penis to stretch it and bring about erection, or only a limp erection. But also leaky valves will let blood drain away and the erection softens.

While erection is straightforward in youth you can see there are many components – the brain, the arteries, the nerves, locked into this complicated mechanism that can go wrong as a man gets older, compromising his erection.

Erectile dysfunction becomes a particularly common issue after age 70, with a prevalence rate of between 50% and 100% in that age group[48].

Other research shows similar numbers. For example, a scientific review from 2017 noted that a man in his 40s has a 40% chance of developing some form of erectile dysfunction, with this risk increasing by 10% each additional decade[49].

And yet another study found that ED is quite common in men 50 years and older, and specifically that more than half of men 70 years and older are affected[50].

What can contribute to impotence?

Given the intricate nature of an erection it's easy to see how the diseases of ageing can interfere with it and cause impotence. So it's a feature of medical conditions like angina, heart disease and high blood pressure, both types of diabetes, liver disease, thyroid disease, chronic bronchitis and emphysema. It can be a side effect of accidents and of prescription drugs. In a quarter of men impotence arises as a side effect of drugs given to treat other conditions.

---

48   https://pmc.ncbi.nlm.nih.gov/articles/PMC3901875/
49   https://pmc.ncbi.nlm.nih.gov/articles/PMC5313305/
50   https://jamanetwork.com/journals/jamainternalmedicine/fullarticle/409619

How changing your attitude and your lifestyle can help impotence

Be optimistic. Just a few lifestyle changes can reap rewards in helping with impotence. You're not being fair to yourself to expect a firm erection if you're tired so take the precaution of being well-rested before turning your mind to sex.

- **Don't let fear of failure become a self-fulfilling prophecy.** Or let worry about your partner being disappointed affect your performance. By mutual agreement focus on your own sexual pleasure and see what transpires. You may find that thinking of nothing but your own sexual arousal does the trick and pleases your partner too.
- **Avoid worrying** by relieving the pressure on your performance. Agree with your partner that you'll not be concerned about reaching orgasm but simply take time to enjoy extended foreplay. The mounting excitement might lead to a strong erection.
- **Taking a bath together** by candle light and with a glass of wine can set the scene for sex. Add in perfume and music and you could find sexual arousal follows.
- **Try another time of day.** Sex doesn't have to be at night and if you feel like sex in the morning after you wake you may find getting an erection is easier then.
- **Be patient** and decide you're both going to give plenty of time to achieve an erection and just enjoy each other's body. If it doesn't happen there's always next time.
- Another option is to **be philosophical** and accept that a rigid erection isn't the be all and end all of sex and just enjoy what you have.
- Remember **alcohol** can lessen the ability to get and keep an erection – "Brewer's Droop".

Impotence isn't confined to old age

It's fair to say impotence is an accepted part of getting older. As you get on it takes longer and longer to get an erection and more direct stimulation of the penis is needed. But with loving cooperation and looking after each other's preferences a couple can enhance the chances of a man getting and maintaining an erection.

Once an erection is achieved, an older man can maintain it for longer before orgasm than a younger man. Around the age of 65 men can take four to five times longer to achieve orgasm than men in their 20s. This is because the older penis is less sensitive to touch. The seminal fluid contains fewer sperm so looks thinner and ejaculation isn't as strong during orgasm as penile contractions are weaker.

Some medicines such as antidepressants can hamper sex and some men may find masturbation can't be relied on to achieve orgasm. On the plus side, orgasm is still intensely pleasurable but after ejaculation, the erection quickly becomes flaccid.

Things you can change if you want to

Older partners would do well to have frank chats about sexual dissonance. It could be an opportunity, for instance, to be open and accepting of each other's sexual preferences in a way you haven't been before and realise there's much to enjoy in your discoveries. Don't find yourself thinking, if only I'd known…

I'm reminded of an occasion when I was invited to a birthday party for Prince Philip. I was in the company of Tessa Sanderson and Joanna Lumley and three of us were there to wish the prince happy birthday in our particular ways. Tessa and I duly did our stuff and it was Joanna's turn. She admitted the Prince was her Mr Darcy and she'd had a secret crush on him from her teens. His reply brought the house down. "Oh, Miss Lumley, if only I'd known!"

As a man gets older he may not ejaculate with every orgasm and that's normal. Instead of chasing a machismo approach to sex, a couple would do well to relax and accept that between orgasms an older man needs to rest. Gone are the days when two, even three orgasms a night were routine.

If a couple adjusts to this, discusses it, they're in control rather than being driven to perform and both can accept this new version of their relationship which is about looking after each other's needs. This keeps their loving and sexual relationship fresh and strong enough to accommodate their changing sexual needs.

Remember, as a man ages his sense of touch diminishes, including his penis, so during foreplay he requires his penis to be touched and massaged and licked for longer than previously. He can always get an erection through masturbation but it, too, takes longer. It's helpful if both partners realise that an older man with a limp penis can orgasm and ejaculate and sometimes enter the vagina.

A woman's point of view – understanding your man

It would be unrealistic to expect the kind of sex you had when you were younger to continue into your 60s, 70s and 80s. The rest of your body is changing so what is on the sexual menu? I'd suggest the menu can be much the same but the emphasis changes. So you proceed more slowly than before. Foreplay is longer than before and more experimental. You talk more and readily give your man feedback about what's pleasurable. And where there are setbacks you're more sensitive with your reassurance and support, suggesting alternative sex techniques. You could find that oral sex opens up a new landscape of pleasure. By the way, you'd both benefit from reading up on what happens to a man's sexuality as he's getting older. And vice versa of course.

For women who want to be good lovers

- How about assuming a more proactive role? For instance, choose positions which give you control so your partner doesn't feel he has to do all the running.
- As we age, foreplay comes into its own. Do what you've always craved and spend much longer on it so that arousal can be relaxed.
- As you get older see yourself as the conductor of the sexual orchestra and take your sex wherever you like, doing things you've always imagined. You'll find yourself in a new world of sexual pleasure and you'll be building your partner's confidence.
- As long as your partner is sexually happy, and you are too, refrain from questioning his performance, instead play up what pleases you.
- There are lots of things that are slower about sex as we age and my philosophy would be to go with the flow rather than resenting shortcomings. Most important, don't let feelings of rejection colour the adjustments you make. Instead celebrate the changes.

A man's point of view – understanding your woman

Some home truths about a woman's sexuality may come as a surprise to men but celebrate them rather than feeling pressured by them. The first surprise could be the realisation that most women can give themselves an orgasm through masturbation. It follows that imitating how a woman pleasures herself will make you a welcome, unselfish lover. Another fact to accept is what feminist and sex researcher Shere Hite confirmed that an orgasm achieved through masturbation is equal to, or better, than one achieved with penetrative sex. So logically, if intercourse doesn't work, you can always fall back on helping your partner to climax through manual or oral stimulation of the clitoris. Most women enjoy oral sex.

It's a wise man who gives his partner special understanding while she's going through the menopause. For starters she may be feeling unattractive but if she also gets sore after penetrative sex due to a dry vagina, she may feel she can't contemplate sex. In this case it's up to you to make her feel attractive and desirable by suggesting you both explore options other than vaginal sex.

Older sex is the time for foreplay and your partner will relish a leisurely approach with time spent on touching, kissing the breasts, tender stroking and stimulating the clitoris. If you haven't tried oral sex, now's the time to suggest it.

For men who want to be good lovers

- Maybe you haven't paid much attention to foreplay before but it's now an essential ingredient if you want to enjoy sex after 60. First of all it's loving and tender to cuddle, touch, caress, rub and kiss and to take a long time over it. Importantly, it'll give an older woman time to become aroused and lubricated.
- If you both like, you can try sensuous massage which is designed to arouse a woman, and you, up to the point of wanting sex, but not having sex. In other words the pressure is off because you're not straining to reach the main event. So you can keep a woman feeling desirable and loved while stroking her breasts and fingering her clitoris so that her desire for sex slowly reaches a crescendo.
- People who have sex regularly tend to have more sex. It's a case of use it or lose it. If you know sex is on the menu your desire for it is likely to arise more often, keeping your sex life vibrant and alive and women continue to have a healthy vagina for years.

- Your secret weapon could be a vibrator. It's a surefire way to arouse a woman, and you, and will increase lubrication too so that the vagina is prepared for penetrative sex if you both want it. A vibrator won't fail to bring a woman, and you, to orgasm, it's reliable.
- After the menopause many women suffer with a dry vagina but of itself it's not a reason to reject sex. Instead lubricate with lubricating gels (water-based and pH controlled) and suggest your partner asks her doctor for intravaginal oestrogen. That'll certainly do the trick.

Sex and chronic illness

Very few of us are in perfect health as we move into our 60s, 70s and 80s. Many of us will be living with chronic diseases such as arthritis, heart, lung and liver conditions. They can undermine our confidence, including our confidence about having sex. No one who's had a heart attack could be blamed for desisting from sex for fear of causing another one. But you can be reassured most doctors would say sex will do no harm and in fact may be good for you. Ask yours.

It's commonly believed sex for people with high blood pressure is dangerous. It isn't. Some drugs taken for high blood pressure, however, can cause erection problems and if that does happen speak to your doctor about an alternative drug without that side effect. Arthritis may cause discomfort during intercourse but all it requires is some creativity to find a position which is comfortable for you both and for some couples it's the woman on top. Taking painkillers an hour before sex can help.

If you can't manage full sexual penetration don't give up on other sexual activities. Physical closeness with touching and caresses can give you both a great deal of comfort, reassurance and joy. Sex toys can be a revelation for both of you.

Caring for your vagina

When we're young we're not concerned about the health of the vagina. We take it for granted. The older vagina, in contrast, must be looked after.

- Never wash the inside of your labia with soap as it'll dry the delicate lining.
- Look for pH-balanced products to soothe the vagina which is naturally slightly acidic. Most soaps and cleansers are alkaline and they can neutralise the delicate pH balance that keeps the vagina healthy and resistant to infection.
- Reject products for genital itchiness that contain antihistamines or perfume.
- The vagina is irritated by douches, talcum powder, perfumed toilet papers and any perfumed bath oils and foams, so refrain from using them.
- When you use vaginal lubricants make sure they're water-soluble and pH-controlled. They're superior to oil-based ones which can promote vaginal infections. They also perish rubber condoms.
- Your vagina will lubricate itself given enough time so extend foreplay.
- Histamine helps orgasm so if you take antihistamines regularly you may have less sexual desire and delayed orgasm.
- Zinc promotes histamine production. Zinc deficiency is possible in women who often go on diets or suffer from heavy menstrual bleeding. Increasing your zinc intake with zinc-rich foods, such as sardines and wheatgerm can remedy that.

Sex aids to the rescue!

Have you ever thought about using sex toys? May be worth giving it a go. Some relaxed couples have used sex aids to spice up their sex lives for years. Even if you were once reluctant, with loss of inhibitions, older couples may feel free to experiment and be more adventurous.

If you're a curious couple I'd suggest you follow your instincts and chat about trying out a vibrator which is especially effective for women, being many times more potent in stimulating the nerve endings of the clitoris than any part of a man. A vibrator is exciting for a man too, you could experiment together and swap notes.

So, don't turn your back totally on sexy videos and movies, magazines, and ethical porn to share your fantasies – they can be a potent turn-on for couples.

Shere Hite

EVERY WOMAN WHO VALUES HER sexuality owes Shere Hite a great debt. In 1976 she published *The Hite Report*, the first scientific analysis of female sexuality. Back then when I read it, it liberated me and a lot of women of my generation from the universally accepted male point of view of female sexuality – that a woman's sexual pleasure is fulfilled by penetrative sex. She proved it's not. Furthermore she revealed, for the first time, that many women get no sexual satisfaction from penetration. She startled the world by saying an orgasm achieved by penetration is no better than an orgasm achieved in any other way and that includes masturbation.

Can you imagine the reaction of a society which suppressed and controlled women by imposing on them the male view of sexuality, not just in 1976 but for centuries before that, taught by the church that sex is shameful and Eve (women) infected Adam (men) with that shame. Truth is women have known for millennia there was little satisfaction for them in penetrative sex. But according to the masculine view it was the only way. Masturbation was forbidden so it was never possible for women to experiment with sexual pleasure from stimulating the clitoris. Shere Hite swept aside all of that and I was liberated and thrilled by the results of her research which confirmed all I'd thought, and informed my view of female sexuality. From that moment on I wrote about the findings of her research so that other women could be free from the male myths about female sexuality and start to enjoy the true female version of sexuality.

As a result of her research several old-fashioned ideas were overtaken by some startling new ones. A woman can have an orgasm at any time she wants by stimulation of the clitoris, by masturbation or by caresses and kisses from her partner. The clitoris is queen. She also revealed that women can have multiple orgasms with no waiting time in between. This is the opposite of any man, other than a young one, who has to wait through a refractory period, before he can have another orgasm. Her challenge to the received wisdom and male assumptions that women are stimulated by sexual penetration, liberated us all and we're still rejoicing, continuing to enjoy our sexual freedom as we get older, too. Even today I see books on female sexuality that totally reflect her view. Her report has stood the test of time.

Shingles

SHINGLES NEARLY ALWAYS OCCURS IN later life and is very painful. It's caused by the same virus as chickenpox (varicella zoster virus, VZV) which has the habit of hanging about dormant in your body, until it's tickled up again. Stress can do that. The rash, painful blisters on sore, red skin usually follows the course of a nerve.

One of the most common sites follows the nerves running along the edge of the ribs so the rash is in a line running around the chest. The first signs of shingles are a tingling and burning in the skin, headache and feeling unwell, as you would with flu.

Shingles is most serious if it affects the eyes and needs immediate treatment such as steroid hormones at an eye hospital. In the eye blisters may form ulcers which will compromise your sight. Shingles of the facial nerve is possibly the most painful, affecting one side of your face and making chewing well-nigh impossible.

If you suspect shingles, inform your doctor immediately as if treatment is started within three days, the attack may be aborted. Eating highly processed foods or drinking alcohol should be avoided as they may weaken the immune system.

Foods high in zinc (red meat, poultry, fish, nuts, seeds, legumes, and fortified cereals), Vitamins A (sweet potatoes, carrots, spinach, cantaloupe, apricots, and various leafy green vegetables), B12 (meat, fish, poultry, eggs, and dairy products) and C (citrus fruits, strawberries, kiwi fruit, bell peppers – especially red and green – broccoli, Brussels sprouts, and potatoes) are all good for shingles.

There's no cure for shingles, usually antivirus medication is used and cold compresses, oatmeal baths, witch hazel and calamine lotion can sometimes bring relief.

Dr Miriam Stoppard

Single Again, Why Would I Not Want To Be?

I'VE ALWAYS THOUGHT MARRIAGE IS harder on women than men. Turns out women and men want different things from marriage and not just marriage, but any long-term relationship. Those differences, by and large, account for why couples fall out of love. I couldn't put it better than the novelist Nora Ephron who said, "The desire to get married is a basic and primal instinct in women. It's followed by another basic and primal instinct: the desire to be single again." Could this be why women fall in and out of love more readily and deeply than men?

An oft quoted study shows women have feelings of love almost twice as often as men. Scientist, Saurabh Bhargava of Carnegie Mellon University in Pittsburgh, published the study in the journal, *Psychological Science*. A second startling result came out of the study, women have a much steeper decline in loving feelings than men, the drop off in women being 55% compared to the much lower 9.2% in men. These differences are even more marked when it comes to a decline in passion, a 55.3% fall in women's desire and very much less in men. It seems the cumulative disappointments with men are at the root of women's increasing disenchantment with their male partners, rather than the common excuse that it's due to wayward men looking for adventure[51].

Men, it seems, are more concerned about the sexual relationship with their partners and want less frustration from their women. Women on the other hand are more frustrated about the lack of

---

51   https://www.psychologicalscience.org/news/gender-inequities-are-important-why-couples-fall-out-of-love.html

communication and the unequal division of chores. One study claims resentment about women having to perform most of the household chores is followed by lower sexual desire due to frustration over kitchen inequality[52]. As resentments build I'm reminded of that gorgeous Stephen Sondheim song, 'Every Day a Little Death', from the musical *A Little Night Music*, as minor frustrations chip away at love and sexual desire.

Another female resentment arises from childcare and it's not just down to parents doing their equal share of childcare, but because of the way children reshape the relationship between their mother and father. I find it quite alarming that men feel less love for their partner when in the company of their children. The truth is men who are loving, caring, hands-on dads tend to have a lower sex drive, probably because of low testosterone but also because love for their children can go a long way to satisfy a man's desire to love and be loved. When loving feelings begin to lessen, it's important to talk frankly to each other and understand the other's position so that resentments don't build.

Many women start off with a romantic view of living with a male partner but find it's less satisfying than they imagined. It's at this point, when a woman realises that her expectations are failed by reality, that she has the desire to leave the marriage. With others, however, there's acceptance. This dutiful acceptance reminds me of something that my mother used to repeat to me throughout my childhood when I was trying to escape responsibility for something: "You've made your bed, now you lie in it". This idea of female acceptance of a less than perfect marriage goes back a long way and was only changed in the early 20th century by World War One. In 1914, women, by dint of necessity, entered the workforce after their menfolk had gone to war. About the same time, the number of women seeking divorce began to rise, and this was

---

52   https://pmc.ncbi.nlm.nih.gov/articles/PMC9483460/

almost certainly because women became financially independent and no longer had a need to stay in a barren marriage.

We also know that women with a university education are more likely to seek divorce because they know they can take care of themselves. But women who are seeking divorce, and the figure stands at 62% of all divorces in the UK, desire to be independent and to find the answer to their emotional needs. It's established that women have a higher EQ (emotional intelligence) than men and may find marriage doesn't cater for their emotional needs[53]. It's a fact that women gain fewer emotional benefits from marriage than men who, in the main, are looking for marital perks. Women get a great deal of emotional support from their girlfriends. Men, on the other hand, rarely have a group of close men friends. Indeed, one in six men don't have any. These days women feel they have less to lose when they divorce because they get custody of their children most of the time, and despite lower financial means and the stress of being a single mother, only one in three women regret divorce.

I remember long ago when I was a teenager and pre-university, I decided I must find enough work to be financially independent. Then I'd have sufficient funds to escape an abusive marriage taking my children with me and keeping a roof over our heads and enough food to eat.

Sleep

NO ONE COULD SAY SLEEP is unimportant. In fact the opposite. The truth is we need less and less sleep as we get older. It gets more and more difficult to stay asleep, with people

---

53   https://cy.ons.gov.uk/peoplepopulationandcommunity/birthsdeathsand-marriages/divorce/bulletins/divorcesinenglandandwales/2019

in their 70s, 80s and 90s sometimes managing on as little as four hours a night. Sleep, however, is so important that most people who get only a few hours at night are taking daytime naps to make up the deficit. My advice would be, if you feel like napping, nap. Our Mediterranean neighbours have been doing this for years, the siesta, sacred in hot countries after the midday meal. The siesta is good for your health, for your heart, for your mood and for your brain. I see only benefits of this downtime in the middle of the day, sometimes called a power nap.

Big tech companies such as Facebook, Samsung and Google allow their employees to power nap during work hours. Why? Because it can improve performance, boost memory and even help ease stress. So, what's a power nap? It's a short burst of sleep, not necessarily an afternoon nap. Just 15-30 minutes seems to be the optimal time to make you feel refreshed and alert. Remember, with power napping there is no 'one size fits all'. Some people benefit from it, others don't, finding naps make it even harder to sleep at night.

Obsessing about sleep, however, can work against us. If, at night, sleep escapes you, try not to get worked up about the hours slipping by. Instead relish just resting, thinking of pleasant things, visualising a lovely memory. Or try my favourite, lie completely still. This is a trick I taught to myself when I was in the throes of a severe migraine headache where any movement no matter how small made the headache worse. If you're feeling tired all the time but are getting enough sleep see your doctor for tests to find out if you're anaemic.

In the past couple of decades we've discovered just what sleep can do for us or put another way, how disrupted sleep (junk sleep) can harm us. It's now known for instance that our appetite hormones – feeling hungry (ghrelin) and feeling satisfied (leptin) are affected by sleep. Sleeplessness results in a rise in ghrelin, the hunger hormone, and you might find the urge to eat is difficult to ignore the following day. Ultimately this overeating will put on weight which is why poor sleep is linked to obesity. I've always considered sleep essential, like an essential vitamin, ever since I was holding down a full-time job while looking after two sleepless babies. I ended up sleeping in a camp bed alongside their cots!

In my experience, dropping off is helped by a sleep ritual and I try to stick to mine each night if I can. It's simple. I don't look at my phone after 9pm, I catch up on the newspaper (I like reading a paper, not a screen), I may watch non-fiction TV (I get upset by violence and bloodshed) such as David Attenborough, anything on ancient Egypt, whales, animals, anything about the cosmos.

Around 10pm I'll take some melatonin – a sleep hormone that the body makes naturally at night. It's gentle and I would recommend it but it's only available on prescription in the UK. If I've had a difficult day I go to bed around midnight where I shut down by reading, usually fiction, classical and modern, in my low-lit bedroom. There's something else you might want to think about, sleep hygiene. No, I don't mean showering before bed, I mean making the environment in your bedroom sleep-ready – low lighting, comfortable temperature, good air supply, no interfering sound, chill out music if that's your thing. I find listening to music on headphones induces sleep. You may like to try white noise.

Tips on how to sleep better

Keep to the same pattern of bedtime
Your body loves structure and thrives on repetition so going to bed and waking up at the same time every day (even at weekends) will help. It sets your body clock.

Give yourself time to wind down
Some people need a routine before getting to bed to switch off their

brain. It could be something as simple as a hot bath or reading a few pages of a book.

A sleep diary can help
Write down what you do before you go to bed and cut out the bad habits like drinking alcohol or watching a movie on your phone.

Your bedroom should beckon you
We spend a third of our lives sleeping so it's important that your bedroom and your bed feel cosy. Have a mattress that feels most comfortable for you and choose a bedlinen colour that's soothing. Block out any light and keep your room cool.

Be relaxed about bedtime
Going to bed earlier in hope that you'll fall asleep won't work, you'll be lying in bed wide awake. Stick to your routine.

How I put myself to sleep when I'm anxious

During a busy day my mind concentrates on the tasks in hand but when I'm in bed it's a different matter. There's nothing to distract me, it's just me and my thoughts and sometimes negative thoughts. So when this happens, instead of lying in bed waiting for sleep to find me, I proactively chase sleep. This is what I do.

First, I calm my heart. I do that with something called "box breathing", or slow breathing. I visualise a box as I breathe in for the count of five, going up from the bottom left corner to the top left corner, hold it for five seconds, going from the top left corner to the top right corner, then breathe out for five, going from the top right corner to the bottom right corner, and finally hold it again for five seconds, going from the bottom right corner to the bottom left corner. I keep repeating it until my heart rate slows down.

Then I relax my body, starting with my toes and feet, going up my calves and thighs, continuing to relax my bottom and torso, moving onto my arms and fingers, my shoulders, up my neck and finally my jaw.

Now that my breathing is under control and my body is relaxed it's time for putting the negative thoughts out of my head. If it's a small but annoying problem that can be dealt with the next day I just keep repeating "It's tomorrow's problem! It's tomorrow's problem!" until I fall asleep without letting that thought enter my head.

If, however, the problem is serious and takes time and effort to sort out, I play a mind game to help me fall asleep. It goes like this: I choose a word, "beach", for example. It's advisable to pick a word that has no repeat vowels or consonants, you'll see in a second why.

Then you have to find words starting with each letter of your chosen word. The trick is to be very quick, come up with the next word as soon as you've thought of one, like a quick fire round. The aim, again, is not letting negative thoughts seep into your mind. Once you run out of words for that letter move onto the next.

So, B – bucket, brows, behind, beloved, bee, better, benign. E – eleven, enormous, epic, erode, elegance, equal, eggs, Emma and on and on. It doesn't have to make sense – it just has to be the correct letter and it has to be quick.

You'll notice that you keep messing up as you're moving closer and closer to sleep. Just keep going. If you run out of letters before you fall asleep, pick a new word. It takes a little while for your brain to catch on what you're trying to do but after a couple of tries it will play along and eventually you'll fall asleep.

Smoking

I HAVE NO DESIRE TO PRESSURE you to stop smoking. If, however, you want to quit there follows some info which may help you. In any case we know people can't be helped, not even by hypnosis and acupuncture, unless they want to quit smoking. I gave up smoking myself 40 years ago. The minute you quit you have a lower risk of dying from a heart attack, bronchitis, emphysema, lung cancer and several other cancers such as bladder cancer. This holds true at any age as we get older. I can't think of another single step which is as powerful in improving your health as giving up smoking even if you're in your 90s. Maybe you feel that you're quite healthy but as a smoker you're not. Crucially cigarette smoking interferes with the absorption of oxygen from your every breath and thence with the health of every organ in your body. In 2022, the smoking prevalence among adults aged 65 and over in the UK was 8.3%. This is the lowest prevalence among all age groups, with those aged 25 to 34 having the highest (16.3%)[54].

If you want to quit and can't decide between cold turkey or stopping slowly, choose a way that suits you and do it in steps. That way you're more likely to succeed. Before you quit, start keeping a daily diary, noting every time you smoke a ciggie, what you were doing and how much you wanted it. It'll give you a reality check on your smoking habit. You'll find there are only about seven or eight ciggies which really matter to you. To begin with, concentrate on these. You'll beat the tough cigarettes by changing the situation where you crave a ciggie or by moving them to a different room so you have to fetch them. Boost your willpower by signing a contract to quit with a friend, with a partner, even with one of

---

54   https://www.ons.gov.uk/

your grown-up children. You won't be sorry. By the way, if you fail you give £500 to ASH the anti-smoking charity[55].

This is how you'll benefit from not smoking...

- The good stuff starts instantly. From the moment you give up smoking, your body will be healing itself. You're likely to suffer from fewer colds, and when you do, they'll clear up a lot more quickly.
- You live five minutes longer for every cigarette you don't smoke.
- If you have angina (heart pain) you'll be able to keep it at bay for longer.
- You lower your risk of ever getting bronchitis, emphysema, peptic ulcer, cancer of the lung, and heart disease.
- Your fitness will sky rocket. Walking, hiking, swimming and playing tennis is automatically on the menu, giving your family the chance to join in.
- Your breathing will be easier.
- Your smoker's cough will disappear in a few weeks.
- You'll be nice to know as you don't smell of stale smoke.
- If you're a contact lens wearer you can keep them in for longer.
- Food is more enjoyable because your sense of taste has recovered.
- No more messy ash trays or stale smell in your car, house and office.
- You save money.
- You're more attractive. Your fingers and teeth will no longer be stained with nicotine.
- It's a real achievement to stop smoking and you should be proud of what you've done.

---

[55] https://ash.org.uk/

- Bear in mind that when you give up smoking you're setting a great example to the younger members of your family, who will see it as an achievement and they're less likely to smoke themselves.

How to stop smoking

Years ago I did a BBC TV series about how to stop smoking (*Quit Smoking*). Remarkably, it's still relevant.

As a prelude to quitting, tell your friends you're giving up and ask them not to offer you cigarettes. Even if you've tried before and failed, think positive and believe you're really going to do it this time.

- Make a plan to quit smoking.
- Make a promise, set a date and stick to it.
- Identify when you crave cigarettes. Remember a craving lasts only five minutes so make a list of ways to deal with those five minutes.
- Get some stop smoking support: If friends or family members want to give up too, suggest to them that you quit together.
- Sign a contract with a friend or family member.

Visit www.nhs.uk/smokefree.

Snoring/Sleep Apnoea

MOST OF US HAVE LAIN sleepless next to a partner who snores through the night. Many of us will have tried to turn over that partner onto their side in an attempt to stop them snoring. And a few of us will have found their partner's snoring so difficult to deal with that the only solution for you, and them, is to move into another bedroom. The sound of snoring is due to the intake of breath causing the uvula (the part of the throat you see hanging down when you open your mouth wide) and soft airways to vibrate. The sound of the vibrations can sometimes be heard throughout the house. They're loud.

Snoring is not a joke and should always be taken seriously, especially in older people. Why? Because snoring is often accompanied by a condition called sleep apnoea. The word apnoea is Greek in origin and means "without breath" and that's exactly what it is. Someone suffering from it can have quite long gaps in their breathing when breathing actually stops. It's due to your airways becoming relaxed and narrow when you're sleeping and it's linked to being overweight and getting on. It can actually obstruct your airways and is often called obstructive sleep apnoea. Sufferers commonly make noises as though they're gasping for breath or choking. Another key sign is feeling very tired in the morning because sleep has been so badly interrupted. The problem arises when the apnoea (stopping breathing) results in blood oxygen sinking. That really isn't good for your heart and brain.

If your partner notices that your breathing seems to stop during the night or you're aware of it yourself you should definitely tell your GP, partly because you want to confirm the diagnosis but also for information on how sleep apnoea can be treated. If you have an upcoming appointment with your dentist, discuss sleep apnoea with them because dentists have access to different devices to help your sleep apnoea and you could try them to find one that suits you.

Almost anyone who snores or who has sleep apnoea would benefit from losing a few pounds if they are overweight. And stopping smoking is essential. If you suffer from hay fever or allergies you should seek treatment for those too. You can buy cheap anti-snoring devices from most chemists but you may need more effective treatment including CPAP (continuous positive airway pressure). This machine supplies you with air through a facemask which is forceful enough to keep your airways open so preventing apnoea and snoring. Some people may find it uncomfortable but with a little practice most can adjust to feeling the mask around your mouth.

Social Media, Online & Apps

IF YOU'RE UP FOR EXPLORING social media, there's plenty out there for you to try. There are some websites like Senior Planet Community[56], Viva 50[57] and 60 and Me[58] that offer content specially tailored to older adults. There's YouTube which I'm just getting used to with its amazing library of video content and lots that would appeal to older people. If it's pictures you want, Instagram or family-friendly Facebook could be your thing. For professional connections LinkedIn is your go-to app.

I think I missed the boat with social media and never really mastered it. So in my head it's unknown territory and one that I feel little desire to enter. I like WhatsApp though and the groups of friends that one can make, in my case, with people I know and love and have many interests in common. I'm not a person who's interested in connectivity for its own sake. Having hundreds of "likes" doesn't thrill me because they're not personal. I don't see the point of being connected to people whom I don't know or have no feelings for. I don't see connectivity as a true friendship anyway. And I'm not at all turned on by the competitive nature of some apps such as Tiktok.

56	https://seniorplanet.org/
57	https://www.vivafifty.com/
58	https://sixtyandme.com/

If I were to suddenly find my interest burgeoning for exploring social media I think I would initially look at only one platform. To look at more I would find confusing. I realise I would have to look at several to decide which one I find the most appealing but I would only go in depth into one platform at a time. We're always being encouraged to join groups that are based on connecting with like-minded people. Even this doesn't appeal to me very much because I feel myself to be very well-connected to like-minded people in real life. But of course they may form a useful outlet for those who feel they aren't.

My need for safety would force me to take small steps and go very slowly. To do this I appreciate that I'd have to look at the privacy settings for each platform and I'm not sure that I have the energy, or the interest, to do that. I understand that using a hashtag and the @ sign (which have always been a complete mystery to me) could help me find interesting content and contact with others, the only thing is I'm not sure I want contact with others.

And in the final analysis, I'm a complete dud at anything techy. I have to use someone who is well-versed in the workings of all these social media to achieve the simplest of tasks. And I think my brain balks at taxing it further than the simplest technical activity.

Saying that, I'm on one social media platform and that is X (formerly Twitter). My handle is @miriamstoppard if you'd like to have a look.

Strength

THERE'S NO QUESTION OUR STRENGTH, and our stamina for that matter, weaken with age. Every day I'm surprised by the things I can no longer do simply because I haven't got the strength to do them. I can tell by the fact that my muscles are half the size they were why my strength has diminished. And, of course, my stamina has lessened in parallel with the shrinking size of my muscles. Exercise in any form will help your muscles to slow down this weakening and shrinkage but it won't stop it because so many other factors are involved, like the strength of your heart, the strength of your lungs, the strength of your joints which all contribute to your muscle strength and stamina.

Regular exercise is essential to stay strong. You don't have to go to the gym and lift weights – though a bit of weight training at home will work wonders, you just need to walk every day for an hour or so and to use my favourite bit of kit – resistance bands. They're fun – like enormous elastic bands – and give extra resistance to your workout.

My top tips for using resistance bands

- Resistance bands are versatile, you can use them for all sorts of exercises.
- Before you start your workout routine, always check the band for wear and tear. They can snap and cause injury.
- There's a resistance band for you whatever your fitness level. Buy a bundle of five with different strengths so you can increase resistance as you get stronger.
- Technique is everything. You have to keep the resistance band taut at all times with the same strength throughout your exercise.

Dr Miriam Stoppard

Stress

LIVING IN THE 21ST CENTURY, we're more stressed than at any time in our history and it's particularly true of working women. Stress is something that we aim to avoid, but it has an upside. A moderate degree of stress can be good for us. In the short-term it improves our performance, efficiency, productivity and many of us thrive on it up to a point. I know I do. For most of us, however, if stress goes beyond a certain point we go to pieces and this can lead to both mental and physical illness. So it's important that one way or another, we come to terms with stress in our lives. We should learn to harness and manage it.

What's so wearing on the body is that we respond to stress with the adrenaline-fuelled fight or flight reflex which prepares us to either stand and fight, or flee. Every organ in the body is primed by the outpouring of adrenaline. Our breathing rate increases, our blood pressure increases, our pupils enlarge so that we can see what's frightening us and a clear path to get away from it. Our blood sugar rises steeply, making available a huge amount of energy to our leg muscles.

The stress is even greater because in our minds we know many situations can't be resolved by fighting or fleeing. Our bodies are switched on by the stress, but they're switched off from action by the brain. The resulting tension and frustration promotes further stress, which in the long-term may develop into physical and mental illnesses.

There's fallout from stress. If the blood pressure remains elevated for any length of time, it damages the arteries and the heart. Other stress-related conditions are migraine headaches, eczema, IBS (irritable bowel syndrome), dyspepsia (indigestion) and stomach ulcer, chronic high blood pressure, heart disease, arthritis, asthma and diabetes.

One of the best antidotes to stress is to be active. So take any kind of exercise, go for a walk, jog, play a game of tennis, tackle a chore, even sit down and make out a list of possible solutions for what's causing your stress. But to really control your stress, you're going to have to make an effort to acquire some basic skills. Two of these are deep muscle relaxation and mental relaxation. Mastering these techniques enables you to deal with stress, then you can move on to instant relaxation and imagery training.

Deep muscle relaxation

Deep muscle relaxation is a technique I picked up in the 80s when I visited the Stanford Heart Disease Prevention Centre in California to make a TV documentary on heart health. You may not master it first time but it's worth persevering. It's an antidote to stress, it'll lower your blood pressure and you'll have fewer headaches so you'll sleep better and feel less anxious. If you'd like to try, here's the drill recommended by Stanford.

- Lie comfortably on your back in a quiet place. You can opt to sit comfortably, and then close your eyes.
- Begin by tensing one hand for just a moment and relaxing it by letting it go. Actually *tell* your hand to feel heavy and warm. Move up the same side of your body to your forearm, upper arm, shoulder, foot, lower leg, and upper leg, and right round that side of your body tensing then telling the area to feel warm and heavy. Then repeat the same thing with the other side of your body. By this time your hands, arms and legs will be feeling heavy, relaxed and warm. Concentrate on those feelings for a few seconds.
- Next relax your hip muscles and let the relaxation flow up from your abdomen into your chest. Keep telling your

muscles to feel heavy and warm. Concentrate on your breathing and wait for it to slow down.
- Feel the wave of relaxation flow up into your shoulders, jaw and the muscles of your face, especially those around your eyes and in your forehead; tell your forehead to feel cool.
- Practising this drill twice a day for three or four minutes is better than nothing but aim for 15-20 minutes if you can. Practising before meals or after is the best time. Once you have mastered this muscle relaxation routine you could try mental relaxation.

Mental relaxation

Again, based on a technique I learned from Stanford, this routine means you clear your mind of any stressful thoughts, anxieties and worries.

- Let your mind go into neutral and allow your thoughts to run free.
- You find a thought recurring, say "no" firmly in your head to stop it.
- In your mind's eye imagine a calm scene – such as a river flowing gently through a pretty wooded scene with bluebells everywhere. Blue is very relaxing.
- Think of nothing but your breathing and feel its natural rhythm.
- You should be feeling calm by now. Repeat soothing words such as "happy", "closeness", "caress". Think of the word with a calming sound like "oh" when you breathe out.
- Relax the muscles of your face, eyes and forehead relaxed, and tell your forehead to feel cool.

Instant relaxation for emergencies

I used to do this to interrupt long car journeys when I was sitting

comfortably. But you can also teach yourself to do it while standing comfortably when you're feeling stressed.
- Hold a deep breath for five seconds then breathe out slowly. Repeat this for a few seconds.
- Say to your muscles "relax".
- Repeat this two or three times until you're completely relaxed. Imagine as pleasant a thought as circumstances permit, such as how you love someone and imagine a beautiful scene.

Imagery training or visualisation

I use visualisation all the time to destress. I like using my imagination to break down my mental reverberations. It can be quite difficult to learn, but this version, which a hypnotist showed me when I was making a TV documentary about hypnotism, is easy to practise.

Think of your right hand and make it feel warm. Imagine your left thigh and make it feel warm. Then make it feel heavy too. The next step is more difficult. Imagine one leg is heavier than the other. What you're trying to do is to get control of the sensations in your body by using your imagination and it's worth practising to master it. After that you'll find deep muscle relaxation simple. And the pay-off is considerable. You'll eventually have control of your body and be able to lower your blood pressure and head off migraine attacks and headaches.

Stretching

I CAN'T OVEREMPHASISE THE IMPORTANCE OF stretches as you get older to counteract the way muscles stiffen, joints lose their full range of movement, and the body complains when we exercise. Stretches will go a long way to keeping your body supple. There are also stretches you can do sitting in a chair.

Stretches should never be jerky nor should you try to force a stretch. Do each stretch slowly and gradually until your muscles start to feel the stretch. Hold for 10-30 seconds and then slowly relax and uncurl. Here's a sample of the kind of stretches you could do. Or again go on YouTube to look for some which suit you including:

- Fingers and wrists stretches – help to keep your hands flexible and strong and are good for reaching and gripping.
- Upper arm stretches of the triceps muscle – for shoulder flexibility and reaching upwards.
- Upper back stretches relieve tension in the neck and shoulders.
- Chest stretches for the pectoral muscles, important for good posture and breathing.
- Waist stretches help posture and make you aware of any aches and pains in your lower back.
- Calf stretches to relieve the tension in the calf muscles, which get tight when heels are worn. It keeps the ankle flexible as well.
- Back of the thigh stretches – good for arthritic knees and to prevent tightening at the back of the knee, so they increase stride length.
- Front of thigh and hip stretches – useful for helping you achieve a good upright posture.
- Inner thigh – these stretches are helpful for arthritic hips.
- Bottom and lower back – this stretch helps maintain your hip flexibility.
- Trunk – these stretches help you to stay flexible and turn easily.

I do "sun salutations" two or three times a week to stretch and keep my muscles supple, ease pain and get rid of the "knots" in my body. Any yoga practice involves stretching, so it's good for your muscles.

General advice if you're stretching

Stiff muscles need warming up so walk around for a few minutes and do some arm and waist circles.

Do stretching as often as you can, daily if possible, as it will help with your balance, strength, flexibility, your circulation as well as muscle aches and soreness. **Neck stretches:** gently pull your head with your hand to one shoulder then switch sides. **Lower back stretches:** grab onto the kitchen counter and step back so that your arms are stretched out and your back is straight. Start pushing your bottom backwards. **Shoulder stretches:** hook your fingers together behind your back, lift your chin up and push your hands downwards while pulling your shoulders back.

It's thought a good stretch is when you feel pain but you should only stretch as far to feel slight discomfort. As your muscles stretch you'll feel the discomfort disappear and you'll be more comfortable. Release and stretch again and you'll find that you're able to stretch further each time your muscles relax, especially when you're exhaling.

Whichever part of your body you're trying to stretch, hold the pose for about 20-30 seconds. Just stay still and hold it, don't bounce because you could tear your muscles.

Try to work opposing muscles. For example, your biceps and triceps in your arms. Start by stretching your biceps (open out your arms, so your body forms a cross then slowly move your arms backwards). Follow it with stretching your triceps (put one hand on the back of your neck, with your other hand grab your elbow and gently push it backwards then switch).

If you work out regularly, make stretching a part of your workout with a warm-up and a cool down.

I have a simple routine to stretch my neck muscles which I do in bed. Lying on a neck pillow I shuffle my hands and arms down the bed, keeping my head still and hold it maybe for two to three minutes. I concentrate on my breathing at the same time and slow it down. I'm usually ready for sleep when I release my arms.

Sugar – Beware!

TO MY MIND SUGAR IS evil and I use the word evil advisedly. Why? Because sugar can do the utmost harm to our bodies. While we love the taste of it, it's addictive and our brain can easily get addicted. It wreaks havoc within the body. Without sugar, the world would be a much better place. I can hear you saying, "But I love sugar and at my age surely it can't do any harm?" But it can. High blood sugar levels from eating too many cakes, biscuits, chocolate, ice cream can occur at any time no matter your age. And that's a slippery slope to type 2 diabetes, heart disease, stroke and cancer. You can always fall back on sugar substitutes if you need sweetness in your food, but then again you may not want to use them. Mind you, when a person is losing weight and not eating, high calorie foods like ice cream are invaluable for increasing their calorie intake.

I remember as a medical student when the whole world thought heart disease was caused by raised blood cholesterol, a professor of nutrition went against the grain saying we should be concerned about sugar as well as cholesterol. He was right then and he's right now.

We used to think that cholesterol was a scourge, but it's been overtaken by sugar. The problem is easily explained: when levels of sugar rise in the blood and remain high, the body responds by producing insulin which lowers the blood sugar. Insulin smooths out sugar spikes keeping the level steady and normal. This mechanism is efficient for spikes of raised blood sugar after meals. If, however, the blood levels remain high by eating sugary, fatty food and the body has to persist in pumping out insulin, eventually we become resistant to insulin, "insulin resistance". Once that happens, type 2 diabetes isn't far away and brings many serious problems like high blood pressure, heart disease, stroke and cancer. A major problem with insulin resistance is that it makes losing weight well nigh impossible.

The answer to insulin resistance is to eat less and exercise more. By the way, regular exercise alone keeps your blood sugar levels healthy, low and steady, making you insulin sensitive again. That's one of the reasons exercise and activity are important as we grow older. Cutting down on your sugar intake of biscuits, cakes, fizzy drinks, sweets, chocolate and ice cream will do the same thing but we find it difficult to do because we see sweet things as treats. Controlling your blood sugar and keeping your body insulin sensitive requires a bit of effort on your part but the effort is well worth the trouble. The pay-offs are great and will go a long way to helping you have a long and active life.

What would be a good diet to head off type 2 diabetes? It's the same old story. Eat a balanced diet with plenty of fruit and vegetables, go easy on red meat, include fish, especially, fatty fish and shellfish which contain the supremely important omega-3 fats, eat nuts, seeds and wholegrains.

One of the best-known is the Mediterranean diet incorporating the traditional healthy living habits of people from countries bordering the Mediterranean Sea, including Italy, France, Greece and Spain. The cuisine varies by region but is based on vegetables, fruits, nuts, beans, cereal grains, olive oil and fish. It's tasty and simple to prepare.

How to cut back on added sugar

Sweet things taste so good, don't they? They even make us feel loved. That's because their effect in the brain is similar to dopamine – a love hormone. Sometimes it's hard to say no but here are a few suggestions to help you resist that chocolate cake.

- For your breakfast cereal add nuts or fruits instead of honey or maple syrup.
- Instead of sugary, fizzy drinks and sweet fruit juices, drink unsweetened tea or coffee, water and milk.
- When you're baking add less sugar than the recipe requires. For example for 150g sugar, add only 100g.
- With less sugar in your cake you might want to add cinnamon, nutmeg or vanilla to enhance the flavour.
- When it comes to fruit, if you can, choose fresh. Frozen, dried or canned fruit is good as well as long as it doesn't have added sugar. Check the label.

Superagers

SUPERAGERS ARE PEOPLE WHO RETAIN exceptional cognitive function (thinking, remembering, making decisions etc.) and brain health into old age.

Researchers have revealed that superagers have more distinct brain structures and connectivity than others. It's thought lifestyle factors like education, socialising and being active probably play an important role.

The Superagers Family Study[59] compares the traits of 95+ oldies and their adult children to traits in older people who aren't

---

59   https://www.superagersstudy.org/en

superagers. This is to identify inherited and natural factors that slow ageing and protect against age-related diseases.

One of the most important factors to be recognised in superagers is yes, you've guessed it, exercise, which needs only to be brisk walking as it alone boosts brain function. Some of them are super fit performing professional athletics even after they're 100. A superager might have had a flying start in childhood as a child's brain develops up to 95% by the age of five, so the first five years are crucial. Intelligence peaks in the late 20s and thereafter diminishes, though some mental abilities peak at 40, even at 55.

You can try keeping your brain young by:
- Keeping learning new things, chess, a language, bridge.
- Reading good books.
- Sleeping well, about seven hours a night.
- Practising positive affirmations.
- Building an exercise routine to suit yourself.
- Socialising with a small circle of friends.
- Doing something creative or exposing yourself to creative pastimes, the cinema, theatre, art exhibitions, music, opera.

Supplements

I'M OFTEN ASKED IF SUPPLEMENTS work. I'm highly sceptical because there's so little research, but that doesn't stop around 10 million Brits taking them to ward off illness and act as insurance against possible deficiencies. I believe eating a good, balanced diet will obviate the need for any kind of supplement, given that a balanced diet is affordable.

My view is corroborated by a US study from Portland, Oregon (Kaiser Permanente Evidence-based Practice Center) which emphasises that vitamin and mineral supplements have little or no benefit in preventing cancer, cardiovascular disease, and death, except for a small benefit from multivitamins in cancer occurrence[60].

The fact is the human body isn't equipped to use vitamins and minerals in tablets and capsules. The body is equipped, however, to use vitamins and minerals parcelled into food. One of my main objections to supplements and vitamin pills is that they haven't been rigorously tested to the standard of prescription medicines. Neither are they monitored for possible side effects. As they aren't controlled, some of them don't contain any active ingredient at all.

While there's good evidence that a diet including lots of vitamin-rich fruit and vegetables will help prevent heart disease and cancer, the same can't be claimed for supplements. There again, high doses of vitamin supplements may achieve the opposite effect from the one you want, causing serious side effects like peripheral neuropathy, damage to the nerves in the fingers and toes causing numbness. The one in three people who take vitamins to protect against illness may be damaging their health rather than bolstering it.

What about soya-based foods, I hear you say. Don't they protect Asian women from menopausal complaints? Could western women benefit too? I'm afraid there's no proof that eating large amounts of soya products will alleviate hot flushes, night sweats, and other symptoms such as vaginal dryness, mood changes and osteoporosis. The oestrogen in HRT beats the oestrogen in soya and other plants by the length of a street.

Then there are herbal medicines. Do any of them work? A qualified yes, there's a small body of good clinical evidence that would support, for instance:

---

60   https://jamanetwork.com/journals/jama/fullarticle/2793447

- Saw palmetto as symptomatic treatment for BPH, benign enlargement of the prostate. Some studies show that it's effective in treating symptoms while others suggest it may actually shrink the prostate gland. Promising though they are, the studies are very short and therefore not medically convincing.
- St. John's wort is sometimes recommended for mild or moderate depression.
- Ginkgo biloba – but only one specific version (EGb 761) for possibly improving memory. The research was done in 59-year-olds and most of us are older than that.

Unquestionably, vitamins are most useful to us when they're in foods. This is because essential nutrients come with the other micronutrients your body needs to use it. It's not possible to overdose on a mineral or vitamin when it's in a food. It'll come as no surprise that all fruits and vegetables are perfectly designed natural packages of the most valuable and protective minerals, vitamins and chemicals – phytochemicals.

All vitamins and minerals work best in unison like the voices of a choir. If one voice is missing or too loud, the choir sounds sharp or flat and our bodies will suffer. There are no better examples of this than the B vitamins. Acting as a family they help each other. When used together they reach optimum efficiency and conveniently, they're often parcelled together in foods. For instance, vitamin B1 can raise your mood but not alone. To work optimally it needs support from other members of the B vitamin family, including B2, B6, B12 and folic acid. If you're eating a salad of dark green leaves you're getting nearly all the B family in a single package.

Do I personally take any supplements?

The only one I take regularly is vitamin D, and then only in the months from October to the end of March when we in the UK aren't getting that much sun needed for the manufacture of vitamin D in the skin. But I do have a personal recipe of my own, which I think may contribute to a long life. There's no single elixir of life, no pill, no potion, no single food, no single rule but there's a LIFESTYLE and it requires more effort than simply reaching for a bunch of supplements. To live longer, you have to invest, work, commit and remain vigilant to that lifestyle. Even if my recipe doesn't result in a single extra day of life, you'll have more life every day, I promise you.

- Have porridge oats for breakfast.
- Shun sugar in any form.
- Don't eat fatty foods, except for oily fish.
- Eat fruit and vegetables at every meal.
- Eat fresh food whenever you can.
- Eat fish, especially oily fish, whenever you can.

I also see foods as medication. So I "medicate" myself with omega-3s and vitamin D by eating a small handful of walnuts every now and then. And I get my dose of selenium by eating a few Brazil nuts. I consciously dose myself with a few tomatoes several times a week because they contain the anti-cancer substance lycopene. I make a point of dosing myself with calcium by eating calcium-rich broccoli at least three or four times a week. And a banana two or three times a week keeps my potassium normal.

Don't only tell your GP what meds you take, include your supplements too

Your GP has to know ALL the medicines you take and that includes supplements. Here's why:

Your doctor needs to have a comprehensive list of all your medications so they can make sure meds don't interfere with each other.

Supplements can alter the effectiveness of your regular meds. For example, iron and calcium supplements can join up with some antibiotics, making it difficult for your body to absorb them in order to combat an infection. And St. John's wort speeds up how your body metabolises medicines, thereby lessening their effectiveness.

So to make sure you have included everything, even aspirin, especially aspirin, when your GP asks you, keep a list of your meds. Update it every few months.

Swimming

THERE'S NO BETTER EXERCISE FOR us as we get older than swimming and it doesn't mean you have to do laps up and down the pool. If you feel up to it, that full body exercise would be good for you. You can just use the pool as a really comfortable place to exercise your whole body and you don't even have to move out of the shallow end. Water is buoyant so your body weighs less when you're in water. When you move any part of your body, you have to overcome the resistance of the water and that tones your muscles and loosens up your joints. Pools are warm and soothing. That warmth serves to prepare your muscles and joints ready for some exercise. It also soothes stiff, sore joints. You don't have to submerge yourself if you don't want to – you can go through an exercise programme without going under the water. All you'll need to get into the water are swimming trunks/swimsuit, goggles and a towel. You can start off by being in the shallow end where the water is up to your waist.

If you feel like it, you can swim with a friend or a group of like-minded people. If you're really keen, you can join an aqua aerobics group which is often available at your local fitness centre. But for starters, here's a very simple routine and you can find more online. If you feel like going deeper into the pool, consider getting a buoyancy belt to keep your head above water.

Easy exercises in water (each for one to three minutes)

- Walking.
- Front arm raising.
- Side arm raising.
- Back wall glide.
- Star jumps.
- Leg shoots.
- Raised knee extensions.
- And then you can graduate to leg kicks with a board.

Thirst

I'M GOING TO TALK ABOUT the all important subject of keeping yourself hydrated by starting with thirst because our ability to sense when we need a drink changes as we age. The thirst reflex diminishes as we get older leading to a state of dehydration and all its unpleasant knock-on effects such as tiredness, lack of energy, dizziness, feeling faint and unsteadiness on our feet. So we have to devise fail-safes for that unconscious blunting of thirst. My own plan is to drink two thirds of my daily intake before lunch, and if I haven't, I glug a glass of water before I eat a midday meal. A tip for you to achieve this is to drink three glasses of warm water (with lemon if you like) first thing, with your pills if you have to take any. You need at least this amount as you're dehydrated after a night's sleep. Warm water in your stomach encourages drugs to be absorbed and you get their benefit quickly. My aim is to drink about eight glasses of liquid a day, more if I'm out walking. And to do this I sip something continuously throughout the day punctuating this with cups of tea and zero sugar lemonade. To remind me to make sure I do this I drink a glass of water every time I go to the toilet.

So what should you drink? Nothing beats water but it needn't be water (though a bottle is handy to carry about) because your body counts up all the fluids you drink whether it's tea, coffee, fruit juice and treats it all the same. You'd be well-advised not to drink too much coffee because it's a diuretic and gets rid of fluid from your body in the form of urine. But the body also adds up the fluid in food – fruit, veg, yoghurt, soup, cereal (with milk), sauce (baked beans). You can forget the stipulation to drink three litres of water a day, it's good if you do but it's not relevant to your body's needs which are special to you and not some formula. I'd suggest you keep sipping as often as you remember.

But what if you don't, or forget, or can't be bothered? How does that affect you? There are some serious side effects of being dehydrated. First, your blood pressure drops and that can make you feel tired, breathless, dizzy, faint, unable to walk more than a few steps because your legs feel heavy and are unable to climb stairs. You should drink more if you become heated because you lose fluid as you sweat more. So in warm weather, when you exercise and when you have a fever, keep a bottle of water close to you.

The one occasion I became severely dehydrated was in the scorching heat of the Negev Desert when I was making a TV documentary about the traditional medicine of the Bedouin who are desert-dwellers. When I got back to the hotel I could hardly lift a limb and I had the worst migraine headache I've ever had in my life. It was a lesson in avoiding dehydration that I've never forgotten.

Staying hydrated

- Get into the habit of always having a bottle of water with you or a glass of water on your desk and keep refilling it throughout the day.
- When you exercise, drink throughout your workout. Try to drink more during hot days.
- If you tend to forget to drink, make sure you have a glass or two of water with all of your meals.

- Water is best but you can up your fluids with other low calorie drinks such as plain tea or coffee, milk and unsweetened fruit juices but no energy drinks, too much sugar.
- Pay attention to when you feel thirsty, don't ignore it especially old people whose thirst sense is blunted.

Tiredness

I HAVEN'T FELT COMPLETE EXHAUSTION MANY times in my life, not even trekking in the Himalayas. I remember only two periods when exhaustion afflicted me, the first was in pregnancy and the second is now. In pregnancy, there are many good reasons for a pregnant woman to feel tired, her body is having to work so hard to support her unborn baby and herself. And by exhaustion I mean more than feeling tired which actually is quite pleasant. Exhaustion is not. That's when I'm unable to imagine taking another step. It just isn't in me. When I was pregnant I used to get so tired I couldn't smile. Why? In the first place your metabolism rises to take account of the baby's needs and this uses a lot of energy. Secondly, there's the increase in a woman's own metabolic needs. Her blood volume rises by a third in order to accommodate the circulation of the baby so her heart is working harder, 50% harder, and pumping faster. The kidneys filter 50% more blood than usual. All this makes a woman extremely tired.

So what accounts for the tiredness we feel in old age? I have to admit I find myself saying, "I'm just too tired", more often than I ever have. And in looking around for reasons, I've decided more often than not, it's due to dehydration. When you're dehydrated, your blood volume decreases and therefore there's not enough blood to go around, so to speak. Your blood pressure drops and your heart has to work very hard in order to feed all your essential organs. This makes you feel tired. If you have anything like anaemia, arthritis, a thyroid condition, and disease of the heart and lungs your tiredness multiplies. And of course you just don't have the stamina you used to have when you were younger. You get tired sooner and don't have the same staying power.

As I reached my late 80s one of the unexpected and demoralising effects of my age is that I just can't keep going the way I used to. I have to stop and ask the people I'm with to stop with me so I can catch my breath and the ache can dissipate from my muscles and joints.

I think another factor affecting tiredness as we get older is our recovery period gets longer and longer. When young, you could go on skiing all day. Then as you got older, maybe only in the morning. Then later maybe only a couple of hours in the afternoon. I had to cut down the hours I spent skiing so I could recover enough to ski the next day. Now I find, even though I'm not performing any exercise as draining as skiing (only walking) I still need time to recover. As I approach my 90s, recovery time gets greater and greater. So now if I do a longish walk, by that I mean two to three miles, it takes me more than a day to recover (two or three days) and be able to attempt another walk of the same length. I find these days I think a lot about my recovery time.

How you can feel less tired

As we age we eat less but we should concentrate on nutritious foods that give us energy. Plan your meals out (even if they're just small portions) to include, protein, carbohydrates and good fats. Graze on nuts throughout the day.

Exercise. Moderate exercise gives you more energy. Exercise like walking, yoga or gardening will help improve your appetite, fitness and your mood.

If you like napping, do it for less than half an hour because you might find it difficult to get to sleep at night, especially if you snooze a lot during the day.

To keep your energy levels up, get out of the house and join in activities you enjoy. Being engaged in something you love not only energises you but will give you better night sleep too.

Keeping a diary of the times when you feel tired will help you plan your day and your activities.

Travel

I'M AN INVETERATE TRAVELLER. AT least I was. Even trips I took in my late 70s are beyond me now. Furthermore, my sons have forbidden me to travel alone. But in my heart I know I can manage with a wheelie, a walking stick and a willing companion – as my son, Will, insists. So now I'm inclined to scale down my travels which earlier were long haul, and involved train journeys and car journeys once I'd arrived at my destination. This is because when I reach a foreign land I like to see it close up, going into villages and eating street food.

Now I feel I have to cut my coat according to my cloth. Adventure holidays with lots of sightseeing are beyond me, I'm afraid. That doesn't mean I can't travel locally, and I will, to countries in Europe and see some of the things that I've longed to see all my life, such as The Alhambra in Granada, one more trip to Venice.

I'd love to visit my favourite ski resort one more time, if only to watch my sons and grandchildren come down the slope towards me as I sit, a granny in a chair in the sun, and scan the piste for their descent. Can't wait. So travel needn't stop, though it's much more complicated and takes more planning than before. Especially as it now involves a travelling companion.

One of the travels that's always available is outings with my children and grandchildren – I think it's beyond me now to take out my youngest grandchild, aged eight, entirely on my own for any length of time. But I happily make up a party of three with my granddaughter, her dad and me. So while I may pine for exotic foreign travel there's a lot to do nearer to home. And while fitness helps it isn't a necessity. I have a girlfriend who's just turned 80 and has multiple sclerosis. She's in a wheelchair so few outings can be spontaneous and require pre-planning and carers, even if they just look on. Her grandchildren, now teenagers, still come to visit her once a week and enjoy a meal with her. She's also very close to her girlfriends of which I'm one. She even made a trip to Ibiza last year in our company. This year she's planning a trip to Greece. So if you're determined, getting older with a disability needn't curb your enthusiasm for travel.

And there's the grandpa who's in his early 80s and has what the grandchildren like to call "a bionic leg". He had to have the lower part of his leg amputated and has had an artificial lower leg fitted which means he can keep playing tennis and skiing so that he doesn't miss out on family holidays.

If you're still an intrepid traveller as you get older, there are a few things you really do have to pay attention to and you mustn't skip a single one of them I've learned. In old age it's "forbidden" to travel without insurance. Checking out medical insurance which covers any ailments you may have is an absolutely essential first step. The second thing I always look after is my meds, which I carefully put into a daily dosing box to cover the entirety of my being abroad. The third essential is to make sure I have the vaccinations which are necessary for the part of the world I'm travelling to.

If you're in any doubt about your fitness to travel, speaking to your doctor before you make arrangements is crucial. They'll give you an assessment of whether you're fit to travel and if their opinion is you're not, you best stay at home. If you're single and in the 80+ age range you might seriously consider taking along a companion who's fitter, younger and stronger than you are. To my mind, a grown up grandchild is ideal, if they're willing. Choose your destination carefully. Anything mountainous is out of the question and even climbing from your cruise ship up a hill to see an ancient Greek temple may be beyond you. Try not to exaggerate your capabilities. Be realistic. Some of the things you used to do on your travels are out of your league. It's wise to throttle back on your adventurousness.

As far as clothes go, I'm now at an age where I'm prepared to travel with the minimum, not the maximum as I used to, and I plan my wardrobe in terms of layers. Most importantly, comfortable shoes. I leave all the glamour behind. On the journey itself I make sure I have plenty of time. I'm too old to get anxious over reaching the airport on time. I don't mind hanging about, waiting for a train or a plane. If it's possible during your journey, take short walks, even if it's only up and down the aisle of the plane or train. And if you're concerned, wear elastic stockings to keep your circulation going. My recipe would be to go steadily and stay vigilant, ask for help as soon as it's necessary. And choose an aisle seat.

U

UV Skin Protection

YES, THE SUNSHINE MAKES US feel better and we like the look of tanned skin, plus vitamin D is made in skin exposed to sunlight. But there the benefits stop and the downsides are considerable. Sunshine contains ultraviolet radiation (UVR) and both its forms, A and B are destructive and dangerous. I didn't know how destructive till, as a junior doctor, my Professor of Dermatology demoed to me the difference between the skin on the back of a baby's hand, the skin on an 80-year-old man's hand, and the skin on his backside, the difference being entirely down to sun exposure.

The skin on the 80-year-old's bottom, and the back of the baby's hand were identical when looked at through a microscope. The skin on the back of the old man's hand, however, showed thinning and ageing due to collagen destruction from being exposed to 80 years of sunshine.

The message seemed clear – sun destroys collagen in the skin, causing premature ageing. The answer is to use sun block SPF50 on all skin exposed to sunlight EVERY DAY. Why every day? The reason is, sun damage is cumulative. Each dose, no matter when you get it, is added to the last and is measured in hours of exposure over a lifetime. If you live in a high sunshine area (Australia, South Africa) you can reach a high lifetime dose by the time you're 25.

Whereas in the sun-starved UK you will have years in hand over your lifetime. That's why it's worth protecting your skin from the sun every day to keep your lifetime dose down. And sunbeds? I'd give them a miss.

In the main the most injurious form of UVR is long-wave UVA sometimes known as tanning rays, the UV rays in sunlamps and tanning beds. Remember, tanning is a sign of skin damage, so it's easy to have too much of a good thing. It causes disintegration of collagen bundles in the dermis, the lower level of the skin, leading to loss of elasticity and wrinkles. In the long term, UVA causes skin cancer, the most aggressive being melanoma.

The vulnerability of skin to cancer also depends on how much natural protection you have in your skin. The paler your skin, the less protection it has so you need UV protection from an early age to limit your lifetime dose. Pale, Anglo-Saxon-skinned early settlers in Australia have a high number of melanomas. That doesn't seem to deter sunbathers. I made a TV documentary on Bondi Beach once called "Dying for a Tan" and spoke to many sunbathers who were happy to ignore my warnings.

Sunscreen use

I'm very keen on sunscreens. I remember as a medical student boating on a lake in strong sunshine without taking the precaution of putting on sunscreen. My back was so burned I couldn't sleep for a week. Most people think they don't need sunscreen when it's cloudy. Wrong! Clouds don't protect you from the UV rays so applying it whenever you're outside is best.

What SPF?

Anything above SPF 30 is good, the higher the better. Always buy a broad-spectrum sunscreen, meaning it has UVA and UVB protection.

When to put it on

Apply your sunscreen about 20 minutes before you go outside. And yes, you should put it on even if you're outside only for half an hour and reapply every two hours.

How much to use

Modern sunscreens aren't thick and sticky, most come as sprays. Make sure you cover easily missed spots like the top of your ears, hands and feet.

And remember, sun exposure can cause skin ageing, skin cancer, melanoma and worsen age spots.

V

Vaccination

I'M A GREAT FAN OF vaccination as it's the only way I know of protecting the body against illnesses caused by viruses and bacteria. Interestingly, the word vaccination comes from the first vaccine that was made and used to control the spread of smallpox, vaccinia. I recommend vaccines at all stages of life, some of the most important being protection against childhood infectious diseases through the MMR, polio, chicken pox and meningitis vaccines, plus the HPV, human papilloma virus, that causes cervical and throat cancer, vaccine given to teenagers.

Vaccination, however, isn't the prerogative of babies and young people. We also have vaccines available from the age of 65 onwards. So, for instance, the flu vaccine is available every year free of charge after turning 65, and you really should have it. You may well say that you've managed without vaccinations for the whole of your life so why would you need it now? The reason is you've never been as old as you are now, your immune system isn't as robust as it was and it needs all the help it can get. Vaccination is that help. There's also the pneumococcal vaccine which protects against pneumonia and the shingles vaccine which prevents that painful blistering rash and is available on the NHS for people 70 to 79. There's also an RSV vaccine against the vicious RSV virus (causes pneumonia) which I advise everybody between the ages of

75 to 79 to have. An infection with RSV can be incapacitating due to a serious infection involving the lungs.

Everyone 75 years and over can get a Covid-19 booster vaccination and we should all take advantage of this. I think I'm onto my seventh booster and I have no preference for whichever vaccine is on offer. To me, they're all equally good and do their job.

It's recommended that people with diabetes have pneumococcal and flu jabs at least annually and patients with chronic kidney disease the pneumococcal vaccine, flu vaccine and the hepatitis B vaccine annually too. If you have a chronic liver condition, please take advantage of the pneumococcal vaccine, flu vaccine and the hepatitis A and B vaccines. The latest generation of vaccines, the mRNA vaccines, are particularly useful because it's possible to make a vaccine from mRNA that's suitable against any of the later variants of Covid-19 within a very short time.

Viagra

I REMEMBER VERY WELL WHEN VIAGRA first came on the scene. It was hailed as the holy grail of sexual potency. It isn't, of course. Viagra and other drugs like it such as Cialis treat erectile dysfunction (ED) in men for whom an erection is a problem. These drugs work by increasing the blood flow in the penis thereby causing turgidity and an erection which may last some time. This is because Viagra keeps working for up to five hours in a man's body so some men find it possible to keep an erection for four hours or so after taking the drug. Contrary to popular belief Viagra doesn't make a man's penis bigger nor does it heighten a man's desire for sex. But if it's harder, longer-lasting erections you're after, Viagra and drugs like it will do the job. Drinking pomegranate juice will help to keep Viagra working because it too improves blood flow to the penis. Drinking caffeine is something else that helps Viagra to maintain an erection.

Remember, the penis needs healthy nerves and arteries for Viagra to work. If you're a man of 80 you probably have some hardening of the arteries (furred up with fat) which won't have spared the arteries in the penis. By all means try Viagra but it may be disappointing. If you have a condition such as heart disease, high blood pressure or diabetes, Viagra may not do the trick. In trials, only 57% of the diabetic men found their erections improved[61]. If your pelvic nerves or pelvic arteries have been damaged (by an accident or by surgery), Viagra might not be the miracle you expect. While Viagra has a relatively high success rate of over 70%, it's not guaranteed to work every time[62].

Men should be clear about what Viagra actually does – it increases a man's sexual response but only for men who have the capacity (healthy nerves and arteries) to respond. Be aware, you shouldn't take Viagra if you have heart disease or have had a heart attack in the past, if you have angina or if your blood pressure is low or high. Bear in mind Viagra doesn't prevent premature ejaculation. Another fact that may interest you is men who watch a lot of porn can eventually suffer from impotence and Viagra may not work for them.

Is it safe for me to take Viagra?

Medical guidelines stipulate you should be fit enough to walk up a flight of 20 stairs without getting breathless to qualify for Viagra. The manufacturers say Viagra shouldn't be taken with heart drugs

---

61 https://jamanetwork.com/journals/jama/fullarticle/188737#:~:text=In%20the%20present%20study%2C%2057,improved%20erections%20with%20sildenafil%20treatment

62 https://pmc.ncbi.nlm.nih.gov/articles/PMC1476025/

which include nitrates that go under your tongue for relief of angina.

It's important that you follow manufacturers' advice not to take Viagra with heart medications that include nitrates.

Why? In common with nitrates, Viagra helps expand blood vessels narrowed by coronary artery disease and your blood pressure may drop, possibly increasing your risk of a heart attack or stroke. There are also side effects, the most common being upset stomach, stuffy nose, headache, diarrhoea, flushes, urinary tract infection and changes in vision.

Myth about Viagra

Viagra is bad for your heart. Well hardly. Viagra was created to help your heart! Researchers initially developed Viagra to treat angina, heart pain felt in the chest. A side effect was erections.

Always check with your doctor before taking an ED drug. And remember, there's a connection between heart disease, high blood pressure, diabetes and ED. That is furred up arteries. If you have ED your doctor should assess you for those three conditions, especially your heart.

If you don't get on with Viagra and similar drugs you might like to consider a penile implant or a penile injection to help your erection.

Vitamins

VITAMINS ARE CALLED "ESSENTIAL" FOR good reason, the main one being the body can't manufacture them itself and must get them from foods. While the body needs all vitamins, it needs some more than others, for example vitamin D and vitamin B12. As it happens, vitamin D is oil soluble which means it can be stored in fat, remains in the body and need not be taken every day. B12 and the other B vitamins, however, are water soluble which means the body gets rid of them quickly in your urine. They can't be stored so you need to eat them daily if possible. Some minerals, iron and calcium are just as important.

Vitamin D is crucial for strong bones but it needs calcium, healthy fats and phosphorus as well as vitamins A and C before the body can use it to strengthen bones.

Vitamin D, found in fatty fish, some nuts, particularly walnuts, and essential oils, is critical in ensuring these nutrients reach the bones. Vitamin D increases absorption of calcium from your gut, and it increases uptake of calcium by your bones so avoiding conditions such as osteoporosis. It's also thought that vitamin D protects you from cancer. While saying all vitamins are important there's only one more vitamin that I wish to mention specifically and that's B12.

Vitamin B12 has two important actions in the body. Firstly, it stimulates normal development of red blood cells in the bone marrow and is therefore a powerful protective against anaemia. Vitamin B12 is also crucial for the health of the nervous system, our spinal nerves and the brain.

Pernicious anaemia (PA) arises when the intestine can no longer absorb vitamin B12 from food and it's largely a condition of older age. Telltale signs of vitamin B12 deficiency are little sores at the corners of the mouth, a smooth, sometimes sore, tongue and numbness of your fingers and toes. Clumsiness gets worse too. If diagnosed, you're going to need regular monthly medication with vitamin B12 to make sure that important bodily functions continue healthily.

Vitamin B12 only occurs naturally in foods of animal origin, so eggs, dairy, meat, fish, but you can buy vegan foods that are fortified with the B vitamins.

Answers to some of the most common questions asked about vitamins.

Q: Are vitamin pills as good for you as vitamins in food?
A: No, they're not. When vitamins are taken on their own the body struggles to use them. To use a vitamin or mineral efficiently it has to be in the company of micronutrients in a natural food.

The result is the body gets rid of most of the supplements and it passes out in your urine. But importantly no one eating a balanced diet has need of supplements, unless prescribed by your doctor.

Q: Is it true the more vitamin you take the healthier you get?
A: No, I'm afraid not. Like any nutrient, vitamins and minerals shouldn't be taken in excess. Some of them are toxic when taken in too great amounts. For instance, too much vitamin B6 can harm the nerves in the feet and hands. This is true of large doses taken in a single dose or moderate doses taken over a long time.

To my mind there's only one vitamin you should take long-term and even so it should be interrupted. You can take vitamin D for half a year. It's manufactured in the skin when it's exposed to sunlight. We, in the UK where there's a shortage of sunshine in the winter, may run out of our vitamin D stores because we didn't manage to manufacture and store enough vitamin D in the summer. The usual dose is 10mcg a day from October to March.

W

Walk...

THERE'S AN ENORMOUS AMOUNT OF research showing how good walking is for you, for your heart and lungs of course, for your muscles and joints, and also for your general well-being and mental health[63]. It protects against heart disease and stroke, putting on weight, even cancer.

Don't think of exercise as a competition. You don't have to win anything and you're not competing against others. It's better to pace yourself if you have to walk any distance and remember you're not in a hurry. Have rests. When I'm walking any distance I take advantage of empty benches and chairs to rest for a few minutes.

Don't think in the short term with regard to your progress. Think in terms of weeks and not days. As long as you keep walking you'll progress. Brisk walking for an hour, two or three times a week always produces results and you'll notice changes in your body (your balance will be better, for instance) and your mental well-being will have improved.

As you're not going to strain yourself, there's no need to check up on your pulse before you set out, or while you're walking unless you get short of breath or have chest pain.

Your goal is a fairly easy one, that you can walk for half an hour at a pace slightly faster than a stroll. And that's it.

---

63   https://pmc.ncbi.nlm.nih.gov/articles/PMC10643563/

Get used to walking when you might otherwise have used the car. So walk to the shops, walk to the bank, walk to the train station.

You don't have to be rigid about your exercise but, if possible, do a weekly plan of three walks per week.

For this amount of walking you're going to have to have good, supportive walking shoes. I favour sports trainers myself.

As far as your clothes are concerned, wear layers that you can peel off as you warm up.

One of the things I find really hard to do is walking into the wind so when you're starting to walk, give windy days a miss, it requires so much extra effort and will increase the workload on your heart.

Measure your progress in terms of the distance you walk or the time you walk. Don't try to increase the speed at which you walk.

Having said that, never go further than you really want to. Don't push yourself. As soon as you feel the strain, stop. Now that I'm 88 I have to sit down three or four times if I'm walking anything more than a mile, so I pace myself with sit downs.

If you find yourself getting out of breath, slow down. You should always aim to be walking "within your breath" then your heart won't be overworking. I now find my body knows immediately when I start to walk up an incline. So if you can, walk on the flat, but if not, take even the smallest gradients very slowly and gently with small steps, and stop several times if you need to.

Walking Sticks

As we all know, walking every day is key to fitness and longevity so my walking stick acts as a spur. I feel its support, physical and psychological, as soon as I start to use it. It gives me the stability of a third leg and my confidence soars. A stick prevents falls as well as conferring stability and encourages you to be more mobile and active than you'd otherwise be, so important for wellbeing and long life.

With a stick, you feel inclined to leave the confines of your home, and every second you're on your feet is strengthening your muscles and bones with weight-bearing exercise that protects your bones against osteoporosis (brittle bones) and fractures. For your muscles it promotes coordination and strength, lessening the chances of a fall. But to my mind it has a psychological knock-on effect: you feel you're in the swim, you haven't been left on the sidelines. You feel worthwhile, not least because of your independence but also because you can go out, do things, see your friends, travel with the family and best of all, do stuff with your grandchildren. I can't tell you the joy of having an eight-year-old granddaughter say, as she's taking my hand, "You don't need a stick, Granny, I've got you".

How to choose a walking stick

The length
Choose one that's adjustable for a comfortable fit with your elbow slightly bent.

The grip
Try out a few while in the shop to make sure it fits your hand and fingers comfortably. You can choose a foam grip or one that's shaped to your hand.

The tip
This depends on your preference. The single tip is easier to use but the multiple tip gives you greater confidence by providing a wider base, and better balance.

Dr Miriam Stoppard

Warning Signs You Must Never Ignore

THERE ARE CERTAIN SIGNS WHICH, to a doctor, raise the possibility of cancer or other serious illnesses. Here are some of the main points.

A major warning sign is the appearance of blood, even if it's just streaks, in your bowel motions, your sputum, your urine, vomit and your vaginal discharge.

A painful red eye with blurred vision or halos around lights, especially at night or in the dark. It's a sign that the pressure has increased inside of your eyeball, acute glaucoma, and intervention is necessary as soon as possible because your sight can be permanently damaged if treatment is delayed. That can be prevented with early medical treatment.

We often dismiss hoarseness of the voice as due to a cold but it should never be ignored if it has come on suddenly and lasts for longer than a couple of weeks. It may only be the effect of a virus but it also could be an early warning sign of cancer of the larynx or throat. If diagnosed early, this cancer can be completely cured, so never ignore hoarseness of your voice that persists for more than a couple of weeks.

A special kind of headache with a tender spot on your temple, just above the eye can mean that one of the arteries supplying your brain is inflamed. This needs prompt attention from your doctor and treatment with steroids. Don't hesitate to speak to your doctor as temporal arteritis can sometimes lead to blindness if not treated early enough.

Never ignore a sudden inability to speak, even though it may only last a few seconds, a loss of vision lasting about the same length of time, and temporary paralysis of the face, leg and hands. These are called transient ischemic attacks (TIAs) and means a tiny clot has passed down one of the arteries to your brain or to the retina at the back of the eye. The body is usually able to dissolve these microscopic clots but they should be interpreted as a warning sign of a stroke and you should tell your doctor ASAP as you may need blood thinning drugs.

Also check out the following...

Keep an eye on a wart or mole and check it every so often for a changing colour (darkening), a changing shape, thickening, and bleeding. If you discover any of these changes, inform your doctor or go immediately to a Wart Clinic.

Always report a lump or thickening in the breast to your doctor.

An ulcer that doesn't heal should be seen by your doctor.

A sudden change in bowel habit, such as becoming more constipated or having diarrhoea. Have it checked out.

Always seek advice about persistent heartburn or indigestion.

Weight

BMI

I've never given much credence to BMI as a measurement of healthy body weight. My most important objection is that it takes no account of how much muscle you have. As muscle weighs much more heavily than fat, a well-muscled person may be, for the purposes of calculating BMI, in the overweight/obese range simply by virtue of their muscles' weight. What means much more to me is where your fat is. You can think of fat on the arms and on the thighs as being neutral, it doesn't affect your health. However, fat in your abdominal region, particularly what's called a 'beer belly', and fat around your waist is a much more dangerous kind. This kind of fat is not neutral, it's toxic. It produces inflammatory chemicals which are linked to heart disease, stroke, high blood pressure and cancer.

So it's that fat which we must guard against. If you see your belly fat increasing, it may be time to take action.

There's no question that lowering your calorie intake will really boost your well-being but how do you know you're fat? The answer is pretty obvious if...

- You stand naked in front of a mirror and jump up and down then you'll actually see your fat jiggling about.
- You can no longer do up your jeans.
- You need larger and larger clothes sizes.
- You check your weight and it's increasing.

The truth of the matter is health risks climb steadily as body fat accumulates, and there's no way around that simple rule. And while I've recently seen magazine photos of fat people looking very happy, all claiming to be fat and fit, the truth is you may feel fit, but you can't be fat at any age and be healthy. Health is different from fitness.

You live longer if you weigh less. That's one of the secrets of a longer life. You slow down your biological clock, delay ageing and avoid some of the diseases that come with age and there's lots of evidence for this. The trick is to lower your calorie intake by eating more low calorie foods that give you all the nutrition you need.

What's more, it's never too late to cut your calories and begin to stave off ageing. Exercise also contributes to a normal stable weight.

Eating less is good for your body

I became interested in the Okinawan people who live off the coast of Japan because they eat 20-25% fewer calories than we do and live to a grand old age. In fact they're the longest living people on the planet and I was keen to find out if their lifestyle is responsible for their long lives. Turns out it is and if you're interested in longevity here are some pertinent facts about the Okinawans. They have:

- Lower cholesterol.
- Lower total body fat.
- Lower blood pressure.
- Lower fasting blood sugar.
- Greater insulin sensitivity.
- Lower insulin blood levels.

So what could we do to be as healthy as the Okinawans?

Well, first we could try adopting a few features of their lifestyle...

- They avoid the two main health hazards of our lifestyle – they don't drink alcohol and don't smoke.
- They practise a cultural habit we'd be sensible to adopt called *hara hachi bu* – that means stopping eating at the first hint of fullness. As a result they eat 20% less food than we do or 400-500 fewer calories per day.
- They don't sit down very much. They walk, do gardening, practise gentle martial arts and dance.
- Their diet contains hardly any fat and refined sugars.
- They're not great meat eaters. Most of their food is vegetarian. Whereas we eat five portions of fruit and vegetables a day, they eat well over 10, as high as 14.

- When stressed they don't lean on alcohol or antidepressants. Instead they turn to strong family ties and community support.

How to reduce your calories

Be kind to yourself and start to eat fewer calories. For starters a woman could try cutting down her calories to 1,500 daily and lose weight at no more than a steady pound a week. And a man might try lowering his calorie intake to 2,000 calories a day. Low-calorie crash diets aren't safe for older people and don't give you steady weight loss. Remember, cutting calories can be effective at most ages as long as it's done slowly and healthily. Consult your doctor for reassurance.

With the first feeling of fullness stop eating
The Okinawans practise this habit and it's a useful habit for us to get into. If you do this you'll lower your calorie intake by 20-30%.

Eat slowly
We have got into the habit of eating food on the run in a few minutes. As the stomach can take 15-20 minutes to register it has food in it and to send a message to your brain that it's starting to feel satisfied, you're capable of eating an excess of calories in less time than it takes your stomach to be aware it's being fed. To alert your stomach, start by sipping a glass of water and eat slowly so that you only eat a little in the first 15-20 minutes. You've given your stomach and brain time to realise it's being fed. You'll become sensitive to the first feeling of fullness, and that's the signal to stop eating. Paradoxically, when you eat less by reducing calories, you'll also reduce your appetite, thereby making weight control easier.

Every calorie has to count
The secret is to eat foods that are low in calories but high in nutrients. Fruit and vegetables fit the bill. They have the highest concentration of vitamins and minerals with the fewest calories.

Weight Loss Drugs

YOU MAY HAVE HEARD A lot in the last year or so about weight loss drugs (liraglutide (Saxenda), semaglutide (Wegovy), and tirzepatide (Mounjaro)) and the fantastic results they achieve. They persuade the body to produce less of the hunger hormone, ghrelin. As a result, you feel full and satisfied and don't want to eat. Weight loss is inevitable. However, I'm not sure that these weight loss drugs are a boon for us who are in our 70s, 80s and 90s. If you're not feeling hungry, you may neglect to eat some foodstuffs which are essential for you at an older age, for instance protein, fruit and vegetables. Weight loss drugs also have side effects, one of which, though rare, is liver damage. Others are nausea and vomiting, diarrhoea and constipation. Don't be tempted to go it alone. Better to consult your GP and decide together on a weight loss plan over the longer term, not the immediate future.

As everybody is different there's no stipulated age beyond which weight loss drugs should not be taken.

Work

MANY PEOPLE ARE ONLY TOO happy to give up their daily job and settle into retirement. After all they'll have plenty of time to take up the hobbies they always wanted to, travel, and enjoy doing things with their partner such as going out for a meal together, visiting art galleries, going to the cinema, theatre, opera, etc. With retirement most people have a lot of time on their hands if they decide to give up working altogether. Personally, I'd have difficulty with that. I've worked all my life and I can't give it up now at the age of 88. Work to me is an essential vitamin, it's what I do. If I examine closely the reasons behind why I work, besides being fully occupied by it, I would have to say that it gives my life shape and also it makes me feel worthwhile. I've always been goal-oriented and confess that I'm lost without a deadline. Writing books (which I thought was over in my 70s, but which I have started to do again at the age of 88) recalls echoes of doing my homework as a child. It's something I enjoyed then and I enjoy even more now. I'm sure working is good for my mental well-being and there's a study which throws light on this.

The study involved 80-year-old Japanese men, half of whom were retired and did no work. The other half went into the office or wherever they had worked only once a week and put in a couple of hours, a half day at most. At the end of the study the men were examined for a large range of health markers, for instance, heart disease, cholesterol, blood pressure, mobility, activity, diet, etc. The rather startling finding was that the men who worked only a few hours weekly were much healthier on all counts than the men who didn't. If I ever needed a reason to continue working, that study convinces me. Doing a spot of work on a regular basis has a lot to recommend it. Firstly, it takes you out of your home and into the mainstream, you meet colleagues and like-minded people who provide stimulation and companionship. Even if your output at work is low, you feel useful, and part of the human race. That's very important for your mental health. You also feel "in the swim" rather than being sidelined and that's always good for morale. And of course, going to work gives you something interesting to talk about when you meet up with friends.

If you feel lost because you're no longer working you could offer a few hours of help to a charity where you could act as a volunteer. You'll be welcomed with open arms.

Wrinkles

WE ALL KNOW THAT SUN has a devastating effect on the skin. This is because sun destroys collagen, the elastic scaffolding in the skin that keeps it smooth and plump and which leads to deepening wrinkles. When we think of wrinkles as being age-related, it's not all to do with age, it's also due to how much sun your skin has been exposed to.

Both the UVA and UVB rays in sunshine are harmful and can damage the skin. UVA rays cause skin ageing while UVB rays are primarily responsible for sunburn.

How does the sun cause wrinkles? UV radiation damages your skin cells by releasing what are called free radicals. They lead to inflammation with each exposure to the sun leaving behind a tiny scar.

The scars eventually join up together resulting in a wrinkle. So you can see how repeated exposure to the sun will only deepen your wrinkles and lead to more.

If you'd like to know more about UVA, UVB and UVC rays here's a brief rundown.

UV rays (UVR)

Ultraviolet radiation, which we can't see, reaches us through sunlight. The ageing component is UVA (long wavelength) and it penetrates the skin more deeply than UVB rays. Its intensity is consistent during daylight hours.

UVB rays (medium wavelength)

These rays burn, only penetrate the skin's surface and cause skin cancers. Their intensity varies by the time of day and season.

UVC rays (short wavelength)

Sometimes called the silent assassins because they're the most dangerous. Lucky for us the earth's ozone layer filters them out. However, they're potent disinfectants and are used to disinfect in germicidal lamps.

How to delay getting wrinkles

- Find out about peak times for UVB intensity so you can plan your protection.
- Broad-spectrum sunscreens protect against both UVA and UVB rays.
- Wear UV protective clothing, especially a hat and sunglasses to help shield the skin and eyes from UV rays.
- Protect your skin by using high SPF sunscreens.
- This is my sunshine uniform. When I go in the sun I always protect my skin with sunblock and wear a big hat with a floppy brim, wear a long caftan with sleeves in sun-reflecting colours like white or yellow, and if I'm in really strong sunshine I might put on UVR-resistant clothing.
- Sunblock can't undo the wrinkles you have but will help protect you from the wrinkles you don't yet have. However, avoiding wrinkles is only one of the functions of sunblock, the first being prevention of skin cancer and for that you have to wear sunblock every day, wrinkles and all.

X

Xerostomia, Dry Mouth

(See page 85)

Xerophthalmia, Dry Eyes

(See page 85)

Y

Yoga

I'VE BEEN A FAN OF yoga for a long time. In my 60s and 70s I had yoga lessons which gave me a grounding to do yoga on my own. I still do sun salutation two or three times a week. What I particularly like about yoga is that anyone can do it, at any age, you just have to go at your own speed. It gets you in touch with your body, you learn the power of breathing by concentrating on each breath and I like the concept that a yoga session is one continuous breath. So it's a form of meditation concentrating on your breathing all the time. You feel great afterwards because the last part of the session is stretching. I learned to stretch properly through yoga.

There's a secret to yoga stretches. When stretching ordinarily we're told we should go no further than the first sensation of discomfort. But with yoga breathing you can go further, comfortably, by stretching more as you exhale, so if you breathe out slowly your stretch can extend by several inches.

Yoga started in India about 6,000 years ago and it was aimed at improving the harmony of mind and body. It's composed of special poses (asanas) some of which are suitable for us as we get older. Besides relying on deep breathing and stretching, yoga teaches good posture through the poses where, for instance, you may do a plank and a downward dog which strengthens your core muscles, and in doing so improves your posture, suppleness, balance and core strength.

The benefits which I've already described would be enough but there's more. Medical research has shown that yoga helps lower your blood pressure and alleviates menopausal symptoms like hot flushes and night sweats. And many people with headaches, particularly with migraine headaches, find they have fewer when they practise yoga. As you might imagine, yoga helps calm anxiety and you find you sleep better. And if you're keen to give up smoking and moderate your drinking, yoga will help.

There's bound to be a yoga class in your locality so seek it out and join in or if you want to do yoga on your own you can get a teacher to visit your house.

Z

Zenith

THE CONVENTIONAL VIEW OF GETTING older is a gradual dwindling into old age, an old age that shrinks from being active, engaged and a participant, to being an observer on the sidelines. If we're not careful invisibility creeps up on us.

Old age is seen as a closing down and if we don't pay attention we shall close down simply because staying in the swim takes so much effort and energy, which are in increasingly short supply as we get on. That's fine if you see getting older like that. I don't. As best I can I want to stay in the swim and am prepared to put the work in. If you feel like me this book will help you to stay in the swim and not give in to the ageism and sexism which seem inescapable nowadays.

To my mind our older years should be seen as our zenith, the result of decades of learning, loving, living and the acquisition of wisdom. We're mature, really grown up, and can make useful contributions as never before to society, our friends and family. We can shun that outdated image of old age if we realise we're far from being on the scrap heap, we're needed and valuable. Old age isn't our nadir, it's our zenith.

When I first started writing this book my aim was to give readers a framework, to see their 60s, 70s, 80s and beyond as a time when they could aspire to make changes to their lives and make their final years contented, fulfilled years. A sort of last chance gulch.

I'm reminded of a wise old gentleman who was really enjoying his late 80s and to my astonishment he said, "I'm at the peak of my powers!" When I asked him how this could be at his age he said, "I see life as a series of peaks, and we have many of them. We come to different peaks all the way through our lives and if I feel down in the dumps I examine my life to see which peak is the next one. Looking at my life this way I always have a peak coming on." And this book, *Sex, Drugs and Walking Sticks* is my next peak and I have to be grateful for it. My hope is it may be a peak for you…

Acknowledgements

HAJNI DOMOKOS HAS BEEN A mainstay in every aspect of my life for the last 17 years. She has always been ready with sage advice, a fresh point of view, and a steadying, affectionate hand under my elbow. No job has been too great for her and her willingness has acted like an essential vitamin to me. I'm more grateful than I can say for her expert and sensitive handling of my text and taking me through the vagaries of electronic rendering of my book. Hajni has also played a vital editorial role.

I'd like to thank Alison Phillips for her invaluable advice on all aspects of my text. Clare Fitzsimons gave me encouragement, without which the book would never have come to fruition.

My family were unfailing in supporting and encouraging me to write this book and I'm indebted to them. My son, Will, has given me, unstintingly, advice on legal matters.

My wonderful WhatsApp group of girlfriends have motivated me to continue writing every step of the way and, by drawing on their example, have provided me with material for this book, and perhaps another in the future.